Y0-CCC-198

COCAINE

"A balanced, lucid, and commonsense study."
—*Publishers Weekly*

"A most remarkable book . . . thoroughly researched and genuinely scholarly . . . but also well-written and easy to read."   —*Newsday*

"Everything the information-oriented flake freak should know."   —*High Times*

COCAINE

Its History, Uses and Effects

RICHARD ASHLEY

WARNER BOOKS

A Warner Communications Company

For T.L.D., R.E.B., and L.J.C.
—Of the many good people who
assisted the author, they
deserve special mention.

Contents

Preface—A note on the author's biases   9

On Footnotes—Or that of which no reader need be
          alarmed   11

Chapters
1. Before Cocaine There Was Coca   13

2. Discovery and Popularization of a New Wonder
          Drug   31

3. The Great Boom   50

4. The Making of An "Especially Dangerous
          Drug"   69

5. The People's Friend Becomes the Rich Man's
          High   97

6. The Great Drought   119

7. Caveat Emptor, or The Way Things Are Now and
          Methods of Testing Cocaine   143

8. The Effects of Cocaine   164

Appendices
I.   Summary of Arguments Used to Support the
          Proposition that Cocaine is Not an Addic-
          tive, Especially Dangerous Drug   186

II.   The Legal Situation   190

III. Do Our Drug Laws Discourage the Use of Illicit Drugs?   202

IV. The Refining of Cocaine   205

V. Storing Cocaine   209

VI. Signs of, and Treatment for, Acute Toxic Reactions   211

VII. Additional Methods of Determining the Purity of Cocaine   213

VIII. Weights and Measures   215

IX. A Cocaine Chronology   217

Selected Bibliography   222

Footnotes   225

Index   248

Preface—
A note on
the author's biases

The reader deserves to know something of the author's biases. Here, then, are a few of mine. First, I believe that drug experts are as given to selecting facts which support their prejudices and ignoring those which don't as are nonexperts. Second, I am not impressed by authoritative statements which either contradict my own experience, ignore history, or abuse common sense. And third, I strongly believe that illicit drugs should be legalized and controlled in the way alcohol is regulated.

In a previous book I presented arguments for this last proposition, and I have neither read not seen anything since then to make me alter my views. Indeed the history of our narcotics laws makes it abundantly clear that the prohibitions against certain drugs have not only failed to stop their use, but have actively promoted it. Our drug laws do not prevent what they are designed to prevent, they encourage it. As one wise commentator has written, they have "had the sole practical result of protecting the peddlar's market, artificially inflating his prices, and keeping his profits fantastically high."[1] And they do a great deal more: they imprison and blight the lives of the tiny minority of illicit drug users who are apprehended; they cost the taxpayer billions of dollars far better spent elsewhere; they corrupt our police officers and politicians; and the hypocrisy with which the proponents and enforcers of these laws defend and support their actions has more than a little to do with the widespread distrust of the police and the political process endemic among the young and minority groups.

What follows, however, is not a book on the evils of our drug laws. To be sure, anything dealing with illicit drugs must touch on this subject, but the primary focus here is the story of cocaine—a drug less understood and more misrepresented than any in the illicit pharmacopoeia.

On Footnotes—or that of which no reader need be alarmed

Most readers become vaguely depressed when confronted with little numbers strewn all over the pages of a book. They are unpleasantly reminded of textbooks and feel that such a production is likely to be dull and ponderous, the work of an author too timorous to write a word not consecrated by the authority of the ages. At best, they feel it is a work for scholars, not for the general reader.

Well, this book is awash in footnotes and *is* intended for the general reader. Why then all the footnotes? Simply put, they are a courtesy to, and a convenience for, the reader. Much of what I have to say contradicts accepted views, and it is only fair that the reader be told where I got my information.

For example, most people who read this book will have known for some time that cocaine is a dangerous, addicting drug. I flatly state that it is not—and the footnotes give the sources upon which my opinion is based. The reader can, if so inclined, check them out and see whether I am lying or misrepresenting the issue.

And that is all a footnote is. It is not a *guarantee* of truth; there are no such guarantees in this world. Nor is it necessary to the understanding of anything that is said. It is nothing more than a reference to the sources of fact, true or untrue. You can check one or all, or ignore one or all. What I have to say is in the book, not the footnotes.

1

Before Cocaine There Was Coca

According to the seventeenth-century English philosopher, Thomas Hobbes, the lives of men who lived without the benefit of a strong, despotic government were nasty, brutish, and short. Their condition improved, he claimed, when they had the good sense to submit themselves to an all-powerful monarch. But not sufficiently, as the record of history shows. For despotic governments existed long before and long after the time of Hobbes, and whether men lived under them or not, they have never seemed fully content with their lot. Even when under the most benevolent of dictators, or when under no discernible form of government at all, people still experienced anxiety, fatigue, and pain. And, of course, boredom— that vague discontent with the way things are. To relieve these symptoms, we have from the earliest times used drugs from a wide variety of plants. The only culture known not to have done this was that of the Eskimo. Not being able to grow anything on their frozen turf, the Eskimo had to await the arrival of the white man and his alcohol.[1]

And just as the Eskimo had to wait for alcohol to be brought to them, so the citizens of Western Europe had to wait until the great series of explorations undertaken in the fifteenth and sixteenth centuries to go beyond alcohol. Until then alcohol had to serve every consciousness-altering need. It was tranquilizer, sedative, and intoxicant all squeezed into one bottle. If you wanted to relax after a hard day, you took a drink; if you couldn't get to sleep, you took a drink; and if the cares of existence became overwhelming, you got drunk. Of course alcohol has its limitations and it is not surprising that the new drugs carried home by the explorers were eagerly received. Indeed coffee, tea, tobacco, and opium were so well liked and so highly esteemed that they were spread around the world with an evangelical zeal.

Not everyone's need to occasionally alter his state of mind was strong enough to overcome the natural suspicion of foreign products. Many felt morally outraged by the introduction of alien intoxicants to their culture. And while a small minority of critics simply felt that the negative effects of each new substance outweighed the positive ones, most confused objective criteria with simple prejudice and moral passion. One example from a later period should sufficiently illustrate this confusion: we know that nicotine is a harmful drug, but long before modern science established a definite correlation between nicotine intake and a number of lung diseases, it was well known that the use of tobacco had deleterious physical effects. Yet the critics of tobacco usually referred to its *moral* ill effects. When Victorian novelists wished to indicate a young man might come to no good end, they frequently pictured him as being addicted to the pleasures of cigar smoking.[2] And Louis Lewin, an eminent pharmacological authority writing in 1924, maintained in all seriousness that:

"The juvenile female flower of the nation, the

14

'Emancipata femans vulgaris' [his term for the feminists of the day], who should bear fruit in time to come . . . frequently fails to do so because the foolish consumption of cigarettes has impregnated the sexual organs with smoke and nicotine and keeps them in a state of irritation and inflammation. Such women, as vestals of the home, should nourish a fire of a very different sort, for their mouth is ordained for other things than to be transformed into a smoking chimney and to smell of tobacco."[3]

Lewin here presents a brew composed of equal parts of scientific ignorance and moral outrage. In the literature of psychoactive drugs this is not an uncommon mixture. With few exceptions, most of the criticism of marijuana, the more potent psychedelics, and cocaine has been concocted from the same ingredients. The only significant difference between Lewin on tobacco and the modern authorities on most of the illicit drugs is that the moderns have taken great pains to disguise the nature of their bias.

A similar mixture of ignorance and moral hauteur played an important role in the long delay between the time Europeans first became acquainted with cocaine—in the form of coca—and the time they began to use it. Alone among the new imports carried home from the explorations, cocaine was not accepted. Rather it was rejected as being unfit for gentlemen. For one thing, coca leaves had a bitter taste; for another, they were highly esteemed by the pagan Peruvian Indians—an obviously inferior lot who had allowed their great Inca Empire to be conquered by Pizarro and fewer than two hundred Spaniards.[4]

If the reasons for the Spanish rejection of coca appear childish and irrational—precisely what might be expected from a period not that far removed from the Dark Ages—it should be remembered that our long-standing ostracism of marijuana stems from very similar reasons: in the East, low-down blacks smoked it in "tea-rooms"; in the Southwest, equally low-down Mexican-Americans cherished it; and no matter who smoked it, it smelled like "burning rope," and the mayhem, rape, and murder committed by its crazed habitués was legendary if without basis in fact.[5]

Europe apparently received its first scientific account of coca from Nicolas Monardes in 1565, but Monardes's work is clearly based on that of Pedro Cieza de Leon, a young man who had taken part in the campaign which brought the Inca Empire under Spanish rule. Cieza arrived in South America in 1532, when he was fourteen years of age, and remained in the Andes region until 1550. His *Chronica del Peru,* published in 1550 or 1553,[6] records the history of the Incas and gives accurate descriptions of coca and how the Indians used it. He did not, however, believe in the efficacy of coca—attributing the great feats of endurance performed by the Indians not to the coca they chewed but to the pact they had with the Devil. He goes so far as to say that "the old men of every tribe actually conversed with the arch-enemy of mankind."[7] Cieza's accurate account of the use of coca coupled with his unwillingness to believe the plant had any special virtues is a typical example of the acute observer who, when the time for assessment comes, allows his prejudice to overpower his common sense. And prejudice is a sturdy beast. Writing almost 250 years after Cieza, Dr. Henry Barkham remarks in his *Hortus Americanus,* "This herb is famous in the history of Peru, the Indians fancying it adds much to their strength. . . . They apply it to so many uses, most of them bad, that the Spaniards prohibit the use of it, for they believe it hath none of these effects, but attribute what is done to the compact the Indians have with the devil."[8] And some 150 years later still, one William Hodge, a professor of botany, exhibits like ignorance: "Ever since the accounts of the chroniclers, it has been *generally thought* that the chewing of coca gives 'extra strength' to its *addicts* and dispels fatigue. The sierra Indian will undertake a long, arduous trip without a single thought of food, but never will he start without a full bag of coca. He *believes* that coca chewing supplies the energy needed for accomplishing

16

the normal day's work on the precipitous 12,000-foot trails of the high Andes . . ." (emphasis added).[9] Ahhh, those poor ignorant Indians—to labor so hard, sustained by nothing more than delusion.

But not all those who wrote on coca were led astray by religious, racial, or scientific prejudice. The Jesuit priest, Joseph de Acosta, who lived in Peru from 1569 to 1583 and who published his classic *Natural History of the Indies* in 1590, was clearly a man more impressed by the evidence of his senses than by the dogma of his fellow priests. Regarding the notion that the effects of coca were imaginary, he writes: "For my part, and to speak the truth, I persuade myself that it is not imagination, but . . . think it works and gives force and courage to the Indians, for we see the effects which cannot be attributed to the imagination, so as to go some days without meat, but only a handful of Coca, and other like effects."[10] Similarly, Garcilasso de la Vega, the child of a Spanish officer and an Inca princess from whom he learned much about coca, never questioned the inherent qualities of the plant. The testimony of his mother and the evidence of his own experience showed there was nothing imaginary about the effects of coca. In his *Royal Commentaries of the Incas,* published in 1609, he gave a meticulous account of the cultivation and care of coca, from planting to the preparation of the leaf for chewing, and did his best to convince Europe that coca was real. It was a subject with which he was intimately acquainted, having inherited a coca plantation from his mother.[11]

The Swiss naturalist Von Tschudi visited the Andes in 1838, observed how the Indians used coca, tried it himself, and wrote enthusiastically on the benefits to be obtained from it.[12] As did Dr. Paolo Mantegazza who, after practicing medicine for some time in Peru, returned to Italy in 1859 and published an essay which praised coca's ability to lessen fatigue, stimulate strength, elevate the spirits, and support potency and the sexual drive.[13] And as did Clement Markham after visiting Peru in 1859 to collect specimens of cinchona (from which quinine is extracted). "I chewed Coca, not constantly, but frequently . . . and besides the agreeable soothing feeling it produced, I found that I could endure long abstinence from food with less inconvenience than I should otherwise have felt, and it enabled me to ascend precipitous mountain sides with a feeling of lightness and elasticity and without losing breath. This latter quality ought to recommend its use to members of the Alpine Club, and to walking tourists in general."[14]

But neither members of the Alpine Club nor walking tourists in general took to chewing coca. General enthusiasm for the plant and its chief alkaloid, cocaine, did not manifest itself until the great publicity attendant upon Karl Koller's 1884 demonstration of cocaine's usefulness in eye surgery. So far as I can tell there were two reasons for this neglect. One has already been mentioned: the European's contempt for the Peruvian Indians which led him to view anything the Indian cherished as worthless. And then, from the time of the Spanish conquest of Peru until well into the nineteenth century, most of the coca exported to Europe arrived in such poor condition that it was virtually of no value, its potency so reduced that no discernible effects could be felt.[15] Which, given the widely circulated belief that the Indians only *imagined* the effects of coca, makes it understandable that coca made no appreciable inroads on the European sensibility until pure cocaine became available. It was all very like the early 1960s when some sociological investigators, after sampling low-grade marijuana and experiencing none of the effects described by their students, happily concluded that these effects could be better explained by the suggestibility of the innocent than by the properties of the plant.

Of course all those commentators who felt that the alleged benefits of coca were either imaginary or the product of a pact with the devil were mistaken. Cocaine and the associated alkaloids contained in the coca leaf had very decided effects on man. The Indians of the Andes knew this by long experience. (In 1917, an economic botanist employed by the U. S. Department of Agriculture uncovered two- to three-thousand-year-old mummy bundles which contained sacks of coca leaves and containers for the lime used by coca-chewers to extract cocaine from the leaf.) And both the Incas and the pre-Inca tribes they subjugated had legends explaining the origins of coca. In the earlier version, Khunu, god of lightning, thunder, and snow, becomes angry when the Yunga tribe burns the forests and the smoke reaches the tops of the snow-capped mountains and blackens the palaces of the Gods. To punish them, he drives the tribe from their capital city, Tiahuanaco. They become a band of hungry nomads, but they discover that chewing the coca leaf gives them strength and the ability to cope with the high altitudes. Thus sustained, the Yunga eventually make their way back to the capital.[16]

The Incas, as befits conquerors, give the credit for coca to the gods rather than man. In their legend, Manco Capac—the divine son of the Sun—brings them not only knowledge of the Gods and the practical arts to improve their condition, but gives them the coca leaf, "the divine plant which satiates the hungry, strengthens the weak, and causes them to forget their misfortunes."[17] The fact that coca was termed the "divine" plant has fostered the notion that the Incas *worshipped* the coca leaf. The divinity of coca, however, may have stemmed as much from a public relations gambit as from the Inca religion. The fourth Inca designated his queen Mama Coca—the mother of coca—rightly feeling that in light of the high regard in which coca was held by the people, they would regard the queen with great reverence. And Mortimer, the great historian of coca, writes that during the Inca period the coca shrub was looked upon as "a living manifestation of divinity, and the places of its growth a sanctuary where all mortals should bend the knee" but that "however much the Incas revered Coca they did not worship it; it was considered the greatest of all natural productions, and as such was offered in their sacrifices. These ceremonial offerings were made to their conception of deity—the sun, which they held the giver of all earthly blessings."[18]

And though the gods were kind enough to provide the divine plant, they were apparently not kind enough to supply it in abundance. During the early part of the Inca rule, coca was in short supply—possibly because the Indians who cultivated it kept most of the crop back for their own use—and the ruling class attempted to keep it for themselves. Ordinary people legally obtained coca only as a reward for meritorious service. Victors in athletic contests, messengers who ran their errands with special swiftness, and, one can imagine, accountants whose vigilance saved the rulers money, were all rewarded with coca. A gift of coca was made, in fact, any time the rulers wished to show special favor to a subject.[19] And the most special favor of all was to be selected as a sacrifice to the sun. Sacrificial victims were given large doses of coca prior to the event. "Even at the moment of death it was, and still is, believed by the natives that if the moribund person was able to perceive the taste of the coca leaves pressed against his mouth, his soul would go to paradise."[20]

As is usually the case, however, what people want they get. The Indians who had chewed coca centuries before the Inca conquered them went right on chewing coca despite the prohibition. Eventually, the Incas accepted the situation, and long before the Spanish conquest coca was legally available for all.[21] The Spaniards had to learn the same lesson. Regarding coca-chewing an "idle and expensive luxury" and, much worse, believing its effects came from a pact with the devil, they prohibited its use on the grounds that it was a heathen and sinful indulgence.[22] This new prohibition didn't last very long. The principal object of the Spanish invasion was that of any imperial power, to take what it could from the land and the people. What the Incas had to offer were precious metals, but the mines were at very high altitudes and the Spanish soon found that little work could be expected from the miners unless they were supplied the coca which had always sustained them. Accordingly, the politicians and soldiers overruled the Churchmen, and the Indians got their coca.[23] One suspects the priests were not altogether unhappy at this turn of events. One-tenth of the annual coca crop was set aside for the benefit of the clergy, and the Church grew rich in Peru. As a contemporary wrote, "the greater part of the revenue of the bishops and canons of the cathedrals of Cuzco is derived from the tithes of the coca leaves."[24]

The Andes Indians and their lowland brothers have never stopped using coca. Precisely how many still chew it is not known, but one investigator estimates the region contains 15,000,000 coca-chewers, another says 10,000,000, and yet another estimates the number to be 8,000,000. The most common estimate is that 90 per cent of the Indians use coca.[25] Whatever the true figure, a lot of people are still chewing coca and a number of people are unhappy about it. Like the Incas and Spaniards before them, the current governments of the region have tried to suppress the use of coca.

These latest attempts at prohibition seem more inspired by the needs of bureaucracy than by the stated fears that coca-chewing leads to addiction, the reduction of mental acuity, and a state of apathy not conducive to seeking a better way of life.[26] Since the First Opium Conference of 1909, the more industrially advanced nations of the world have attempted to control the production and use of all drugs they consider harmful to their trade relations and the welfare of their citizens. They have attempted this through international conferences, the League of Nations, and now through the United Nations. And, of course, they have carried on the good work in an even more unfettered way within their own national boundaries—as any user of illicit drugs can testify.

Very large national and international bureaucracies have grown up to implement this objective and, as is usually the case with bureaucracies, they tend to be more concerned with consolidating and expanding their power than with examining the reasons for their existence. The justification for spending tax money and limiting freedom which has always been used by the drug bureaucracies is that the citizens of the world must be protected from habit-forming, dangerous drugs.

But despite public statements filled with pious morality and concern for drug "victims," the true reasons for calling the First Opium Conference had much more to do with business and politics than with any real concern for the welfare of individuals. Opium had, during the nineteenth century, caused serious international problems: two wars between China and England; trouble for the Americans governing the Philippine Islands where a Spanish-instituted system of licensing narcotics addicts prevailed; and bitter complaints by the trading nations of the world that the Chinese were spending most of their bullion on opium from British India and thus had little left over to spend with them.[27] Coca and cocaine had caused no such vexing problems, yet they were included in the protocols issued by the Hague Convention of 1912, because (1) the reasons offered the public for controlling the international drug traffic all centered around the need and duty to protect citizens from the perils of the drug habit, and (2) coca and cocaine had for many years been considered addictive drugs. They thus had to be included among the banned substances if the protocols were to be consistent with the public pronouncements. So at least it seems to me.

But neither coca nor cocaine are addicting substances like the opiates. No tolerance is built up to the drug, and cessation of use produces no noticeable withdrawal symptoms. Indians start chewing coca in their teens and, circumstances permitting, continue until they die—and all observers agree they use about the same amount daily from the beginning of this cycle to the end. Moreover, Indians recruited into the Peruvian Army gave up coca with no apparent difficulty when the army banned its use, as did those who moved to cities where coca was not readily obtainable.[28]

Despite these facts and despite centuries of evidence to the effect that coca is beneficial to the Andes Indian, that indeed it seems unlikely they could survive the rigors of their harsh environment without its aid, attempts are still being made to prohibit its use.[29] Whether this stems simply from the natural urge of bureaucrats to extend their power wherever they can, or whether they truly believe that coca has a deleterious effect, it is hard to say. In any case, the prohibitionists bolster their position with exceedingly dubious reports which claim to demonstrate a statistical correlation between illiteracy and coca-chewing, between lack of interest and reduced aptitude in learning and coca-chewing, and between malnutrition and coca-chewing[30]—all of which imply that coca-chewing *causes* these conditions.[31]

Apart from the fact that these reports are the work of people who evince no high regard for the Indian way of life, they continually draw unwarranted conclusions from highly selective data. And they do so with a dogmatic assurance which makes one wonder about the motives of the authors. For example, Marcel Granier-Doyeux, a drug bureaucrat par excellence— vice-president of the International Narcotics Control Board, member of the World Health Organization consultative group on dependence-producing drugs, head of the Department of Pharmacology and Toxicology at the Central University of Venezuela, and president of the Venezuelan Academy of Medicine— writes with that no-nonsense certainty one comes to expect from the elect, that "The harmful effects of chewing coca leaves have been clearly established by the Commission of Enquiry appointed by the United Nations in 1949."[32] Granier-Doyeux was, of course, a member of the Commission. But the single study he cites to justify the sweeping conclusion of the UN report is that of Gutierrez-Noriega on the relation of coca-chewing and illiteracy, a study which in its conclusions makes the serious, and invalidating, error of selecting

23

one factor in the lifestyle of the Indians and ignoring all others.[33]

The other factors in the Indian way of life include wretched poverty, grossly inadequate diets, and living and working at altitudes where the oxygen content of the air is severely restricted—all of which are known to seriously affect learning ability. To put it another way, people living in such conditions would predictably have problems in school whether they chewed coca or not. As for coca-chewing's being the cause of malnutrition, this is an uglier and more complicated situation. There is a scarcity of food in the high Andes and without coca the average Indian wouldn't have sufficient energy to work. Rather than being the cause of malnutrition, coca-chewing is a symptom of malnutrition. Those governments attempting to prohibit coca would better exhibit their concern for the plight of the Indians by providing them with adequate diets, by attacking the cause of malnutrition rather than its symptom. As things now stand, prohibiting coca-chewing without providing the means for an adequate diet is nothing more than a means, conscious or unconscious, of exterminating the Indians.

Even an adequate diet, however, would not eliminate the Andes Indian's need for coca. Studies have been made indicating that coca is essential to the health of the Indian since coca increases the heart rate, arterial pressure, and the number of breaths per minute —all of which are of great value when living and working at high altitudes.[34]

Not surprisingly, the coca prohibitionists pay little if any attention to the testimony of doctors, travelers, and scientists who have spent long periods of time in the coca regions, chewed coca themselves, reported decided benefits from the practice, and noted no ill effects. A few nineteenth-century reports have already been cited. Here is a contemporary quotation concerning Professor Richard Evans Schultes, director of the Botanical Museum of Harvard University, and a leading authority on the drugs of plant origin used by primitive peoples: ". . . during his plant explora-

24

tions in the Amazon Valley he chewed coca leaves daily for eight years, did not become addicted, and suffered no apparent harm from the custom."[35] Nor do these prohibitionists pay attention to those researchers who have devoted much time and attention to investigating the literature on the effects of coca. Edward Brecher, author of the Consumers Union Report on *Licit & Illicit Drugs,* is such a researcher and has this to say on the subject: "A search of the medical literature has turned up little data to indicate that the chewing of coca leaves or the imbibing of beverages containing small amounts of coca is more damaging to mind or body than the drinking of coffee or tea."[36]

But whatever the motives of the coca prohibitionist and the drug control bureaucrats, it seems that their desire to control what people do is far stronger than their respect for truth. In the article in which Granier-Doyeux flatly stated that the harmful effects of coca had been proved, he also wrote of LSD that "there is no definite proof of its therapeutic value."[37] The fact is that long-term studies of its effectiveness in treating alcoholism and in treating a variety of psychiatric problems leave no doubts as to its therapeutic value.[38] The studies referred to are only those of which Granier-Doyeux, as a recognized "expert" on drugs, should have been aware. Of course, he may hold to the very strictest standard of definite proof and discount these studies as not being definitive. But if that is the case, he has no business citing Gutierrez-Noriega to show that coca-chewing has been *proved* to be harmful.

The root of all this controversy, the coca shrub— and, primarily, the variety *Erythroxylon coca*[39]—is a flowering plant indigenous to the eastern slopes of the Andes mountains. The heart of the coca region is in Peru and Bolivia but coca is found along the entire curve of the Andes from the southern tip of Chile to the borders of the Caribbean, at elevations of from 1,500 to 6,000 feet.[40] It has also been grown success-

25

fully in Java, Ceylon, India, Africa, and the West Indies, but most of these plantations have fallen into disuse.[41]

The wild coca plant grows as high as fifteen feet but to facilitate picking, the cultivated plants are kept at heights of from three to six feet. The cultivation of coca is carried on in small, terraced plantations called *cocales* and, whether in Chile in the south or Venezuela in the north, the cocales appear much the same—small hillside clearings of usually no more than two or three acres. On the average there are about 7,000 plants per acre, yielding four ounces of leaves per plant at the main harvest. Normally there are three regular harvests—in March, at the end of June, and at the end of October or the beginning of November— plus a preliminary trimming operation preceding the March harvest. The first regular harvest in March is the most productive, the one in June is usually sparse, while the fall harvest yields less than that in March but considerably more than the one in June. The harvesters are usually women and children, and four or five expert pickers in a good *cocal* can pick twenty-five pounds of leaves in a day.[42]

The picked leaves are taken to a drying area and spread out in layers two or three inches deep. In good weather the drying operation can be completed in six hours. If it rains the leaves are quickly swept under the sheds that surround the drying area. (Damp leaves ferment, a process that tends to break down the cocaine and other alkaloids.) After the leaves have dried, they are gathered into large heaps and left for about three days, during which time the leaves "sweat." The crisp dried leaf becomes soft and pliable, rendering it more palatable to the chewer. The leaves are then sun-dried for half an hour or so and packed for shipment.[43]

The two major coca-growing countries, Bolivia and Peru, produce approximately 11.5 million kilograms of leaves a year. Ninety per cent of this is said to be consumed at home by the coca-chewers; the remainder is exported as leaves, as crude cocaine or as refined cocaine. The United States is the world's largest importer of coca leaves, buying some 200,000 to 250,000 kilograms annually.[44]

There are a great many varieties of coca, but most of the coca that is used can be grouped broadly into two varieties—the Bolivian, or Huanico coca, and the Peruvian, or Truxillo coca. The legal manufacturers of cocaine rely almost entirely on the Bolivian variety inasmuch as it contains a higher percentage of cocaine and a lower percentage of the associated alkaloids than does the Peruvian variety.[45] The total alkaloid content of the coca leaf ranges from 0.7 to 1.5 per cent, with cocaine constituting anywhere from thirty to seventy-five per cent of this total.[46] (Some authorities list the cocaine content as being between 0.5 and 1.5 per cent.)[47] In addition to cocaine and the associated alkaloids coca contains vitamin C and many of the B vitamins. But since pharmacologists have done very little work in this area, the amount of these vitamins present is not known.

The *coquero,* as the Indian coca-chewer is called, takes his coca with a little lime, the ashes of the Andean cereal, *quinoa,* or a powder made from crushed shells.[48] The function of the lime or other material is to extract the cocaine and its associated alkaloids from the leaf. The coca-chewer doesn't really chew and swallow the coca leaves; rather he sucks on a quid of leaves—as one might suck a peach pit—and discards it when the juices have been extracted. The typical coca-chewer is said to use about two ounces of leaves per day. Taking this figure as the norm and assuming the cocaine content of the quid to be approximately 0.7 per cent, virtually every authority on the subject has estimated that the Indian coca-chewers ingest very little cocaine—something on the order of 0.6 grains of cocaine a day.[49] And, given the fact that it requires 15.4 grains to constitute a gram, this is certainly a very small intake of cocaine—or would be, if true. But either none of the authorities can do simple arithmetic, or all of them have relied upon some long-forgotten miscreant and perpetuated his error. For there are 437.5 grains to an ounce, or 875 grains in

27

two ounces, and assuming the cocaine content to be 0.7 per cent, the average Indian has an intake of about 6 grains of cocaine a day, *not* 0.6 grains a day. And this is a goodly regular dosage by any standard. A typical user of illicit cocaine will snort from four to eight grains a day, and that usually only a few days a month.[50]

This long perpetuated error about the amount of cocaine taken by the Indians is of great significance. For modern researchers who believe cocaine to be a dangerous addictive drug have always argued that the fact that the Indians seem to suffer neither addiction nor adverse effects from the habitual chewing of coca leaves cannot be used to support the thesis that cocaine is not an addictive drug. After all, they say, the Indians ingest insignificant amounts of cocaine, less than a grain a day on average. But as we have seen, they use about 6 grains a day, or as much as most modern users.

Since the remainder of this book will be concerned with cocaine rather than with its mother plant, coca, a short preview of the effects of cocaine may be useful to the reader. (A detailed account of both the positive and adverse effects of the drug will be found in the last chapter.)

To begin with, the great majority of users rarely take more cocaine in a day than do the Indian coca-chewers, and they do not use the drug with anything like the frequency of the Indians. They typically use cocaine a day or a few days at a time and go without it for weeks at a time. There are two reasons for this pattern. First, cocaine is a very expensive drug on the illicit market, and few people can afford it on a continuous basis. And secondly, it is not an addictive drug like heroin, not a drug the user *must* have. A small number of users do take cocaine on a daily basis and in significantly larger quantities than those just mentioned.

What the cocaine user basically gets for his money is euphoria, increased energy, and a lessening of fatigue. In short, the user feels good. The degree to which these effects are experienced depends both on the dose and the individual. Usually, the more cocaine, the more powerful the effects. But a point is reached where more cocaine becomes counterproductive—feelings of euphoria may turn into feelings of paranoia, the lessening of fatigue into insomnia, and so on. This point varies from individual to individual. No stimulus has precisely the same effect on everyone, and cocaine is no exception to this rule.

The literature on cocaine contains many references to serious adverse reactions experienced by users—dependence, depression, paranoia, hallucinations, even death—but all these references date back many decades, are based on very few cases, and in general are grossly exaggerated. In recent years there have been no reports of deaths among cocaine users, and very, very few reports of the other serious adverse reactions. There are, however, a small number of heavy users who experienced reactions which led them to warn the drug community of the dangers of cocaine. The statement of a Jefferson Airplane member is a representative example:

"I stopped using coke a year and a half ago, when it was obvious it had become more dangerous than useful to me. Cocaine is a really great drug, it's a great way to feel good, and you can function and work relatively clearly on it, like for 12 or 15 hours straight, without losing your perspective the way you do on uppers or speed.

"But it's not controllable. It's not that you have an increasing need or tolerance, it's that it's so pleasant you can't control your use of it. And when you're heavy into it, it makes you cold toward people, in the sense that you're thinking of so many things that you can't possibly accomplish them all, and you're thinking of how to do all the things and you don't think about the people you're around."[51]

With cocaine, as with most pleasures, excess is usually less than beneficial. On his own admission, Paul Kantner was a heavy user and paid the penalty for overindulgence. But though he and some other immoderates found it difficult to control their intake, they are exceptions and not the rule. The vast majority of cocaine users never have such a problem. And even among heavy users most are able to control their use of cocaine to the extent that serious adverse reactions are rare.

2

Discovery and Popularization of a New Wonder Drug

Though cocaine is but one of several alkaloids found in the coca leaf, it is by weight—30 to 75 per cent of the total alkaloid content—and by virtue of its properties as a central nervous system stimulant and local anesthetic easily the most important one. Alkaloids are commonly defined as a large group of basic organic substances (there are hundreds of them), usually of plant origin, which contain carbon, hydrogen, nitrogen and, in most cases, oxygen—and which generally have a pronounced physiological action on animal organisms.[1] In many cases they have a pronounced psychological effect as well. Atropine, caffeine, nicotine, mescaline, and morphine are, for example, alkaloids with unmistakable psychoactive effects.

The nature of alkaloids was not understood until the early part of the nineteenth century, and the term itself was not coined until 1821.[2] But, needless to say, people were being affected by alkaloids long before this time. Opium (morphine) was smoked, the sacred mushroom (muscarine or psilocybin, depending on the geographic location) eaten, and coca leaves (cocaine) chewed before the birth of Christ. And all of these dope users knew very well that *something* in their product of choice was *doing* something to them. But until the rise of science in seventeenth-century Europe there is no evidence to suggest that anyone was interested in discovering *what* it was in these plants that caused such agreeable, and sometimes not so agreeable, sensations. Some plants made you feel good, some killed you, and it was enough to know which was which. A marked change occurred in this simple pragmatic attitude during the seventeenth century, when opium was becoming popular in Europe and the new scientific consciousness was developing. Inevitably, these fledgling investigators began wondering what it was in opium that affected people as it did. Or, as they put it, what was the active principle of opium?[3]

The answer did not come until 1803 when F. W. Sertürner isolated morphine from opium and, even more importantly, gained the first real insight into the chemical and physiological nature of the alkaloids.[4] Sertürner's feat revolutionized the practice of medicine. Soon, a measured dose of a pure drug could be prescribed and accurate research could be done on the differences between specific doses. The methods he developed sparked a wave of research into the other plant alkaloids. By 1840 nearly all the medically important alkaloids had been isolated: strychnine in 1817; quinine and caffeine in 1820; nicotine in 1828; and atropine in 1833.[5] Cocaine is conspicuously missing from the list. That it was the last of the major plant alkaloids to be isolated can probably best be explained by coca's lack of popularity in Europe.

Who first isolated cocaine, and when, is a matter of dispute. And, since cocaine is probably the least understood and most consistently misrepresented drug in the pharmacopoeia, this absence of clear answers to simple questions seems peculiarly appropriate. Two sources give the honor to one Gaedkin in 1844.[6] Four credit Gaedecke (variously spelled Gaedeke, Gaedche, Gardecke, Gardeke) in 1855.[7] Three say that Albert Niemann did it in 1858,[8] four think it was in 1859,[9] and five hold out for 1860.[10] In my own secondhand view, the 1844 date is probably an error and, given all the ways I've seen Gaedecke's name spelled, the Gaedkin of 1844 may very well be the Gaedecke of 1855. At any rate, it seems relatively clear that Gaedecke isolated cocaine prior to Niemann and that Niemann did the work independently in either 1858, 1859, or 1860, perhaps obtaining a purer product. Gaedecke named the new alkaloid erythroxyline, after the botanical name of coca. (A. L. De Jussieu had classed coca with the genus *erythroxylon* and it appeared in Lamarck's *Encyclopédie Méthodique Botanique* as *Erythroxylon coca* in 1783.)[11] Niemann called it cocaine.

In any event cocaine ($C_{17}H_{21}NO_4$) was now on the shelf and one might reasonably expect a veritable explosion of cocaine research. After all, the drug had given rise to absolutely contradictory reports for centuries. The positive reports given by the few Europeans who had used coca in South America had been countered by the negative findings of researchers' working, in all probability, with inert leaves. But now all doubts could be dispelled. There clearly was an active ingredient in coca. They had it before them, a pile of shining crystals.

But cocaine, like its parent coca, did not meet with ready acceptance by the white man. Perhaps the generally held belief that the properties of coca were mythical inculcated negative expectations to the extent that few people were eager to devote their time to a probably worthless project. And perhaps coca's paradoxical nature—its reputed euphoric quality coupled with its ability to numb the area of application—reinforced the belief that its reputation was indeed mythical. After all, did it seem likely that what deadened some sensations heightened others? Or possibly the very fact that cocaine wasn't isolated until long after the great enthusiasm for alkaloid research had passed was a factor. Science has its fads. Then too, many of the cocaine preparations were of doubtful quality.[12] In short, with certain exceptions, the early work done on cocaine produced inconclusive results. And the suggestions made by those who obtained positive results were either ignored or not fully appreciated.

As early as 1862 a medical researcher named Schroff put some cocaine on the tip of his tongue and noted the numbing effect, but neither he nor anyone else seemed to realize the significance of this action.[13] Then in 1868, a Peruvian physician, Thomas Moreno y Maiz reported the effects of cocaine upon a frog and suggested that cocaine might be a useful local anesthetic.[14] No one took up his suggestion. So far as I can tell, the early European researchers concentrated on the physiological effects of cocaine and either didn't notice or failed to report on its other properties. In America, researchers directed their attention to the psychoactive effects. In 1878 Dr. W. H. Bentley announced the successful switching of a morphine addict to cocaine.[15] In 1880, a Dr. Palmer wrote an extensive account in the *Louisville Medical News* on the treatment of morphine addiction with cocaine.[16] And from 1880 through 1882, *"Erythroxylon coca* in the opium habit" was a regular heading in the reports of the *Detroit Therapeutic Gazette.*[17]

Then in 1883, Dr. Theodor Aschenbrandt, a German army physician, obtained a supply of cocaine from the pharmaceutical house of Merck and issued it to some Bavarian soldiers during the autumn maneuvers. He reported that the cocaine-using soldiers exhibited more energy and a notably greater ability to endure fatigue than did the others.[18] Given any army's delight in energetic troops with great powers of endurance, this experiment alone would probably have been sufficient to assure the widespread use of cocaine. Amphetamines, for example, were issued for these purposes to the American, British, German, and Japanese armies on an enormous scale during World War II.[19]

Whatever might have happened as a result of Aschenbrandt's experiment, what *did* happen was that Sigmund Freud came across his report at a time when he had become interested in cocaine through the articles appearing in the *Detroit Therapeutic Gazette* and went on to become the single most important popularizer of cocaine in Europe. Freud at this period was a poor, 28-year-old neurologist who, according to his biographer, Ernest Jones, was "constantly occupied with the endeavours to make a name for himself by discovering something important in either clinical or pathological medicine."[20] The motives behind this drive for success were less purely egotistical than might appear. Freud desperately sought professional recognition, but less for fame itself than for the fact that professional success would allow him to marry his fiancée, Martha Bernays, much earlier than would be likely in the normal course of events.[21]

Aschenbrandt published his account on December 12, 1883. Four months later, on April 21, 1884, Freud wrote Martha that "I have been reading about cocaine, the essential constituent of coca leaves which some Indian tribes chew to enable them to resist privations and hardships. A German has been employing it with soldiers and has in fact reported that it increases their energy and capacity to endure. I am procuring some myself and will try it with cases of heart disease and also of nervous exhaustion, particularly in the miserable condition after the withdrawal of morphium [Dr. Fleischl]."[22] It seems likely he intended to dose himself as well—not simply in his role as careful investigator but, rather, hoping to alleviate certain recurring ailments. Freud had suffered from depression, chronic fatigue, and a host of other neurotic symptoms for several years.[23]

Cocaine was to change all that, but first he had to obtain a sample. At this point Freud experienced a moment of dismay, one familiar to most cocaine seekers—he didn't have enough money. It's worth quoting his biographer on the situation:

"The first obstacle proved to be the cost of the

cocaine he had ordered from Merck of Darmstadt; instead of a gram costing, as he had expected, 33 kreutzer (13 cents) he was dismayed to find it cost 3 gulden 33 kreutzer ($1.27). At first he thought this meant the end of his research, but after getting over the shock he boldly ordered a gram in the hope of being able to pay for it sometime."[24]

After Freud got his cocaine on credit he put 50 milligrams (1/20) gram) into a glass of water and drank it. A few minutes later he noticed that his bad mood had evaporated—he felt cheerful and energetic.[25] Not long after this, he gave some to his friend Fleischl who had become addicted to morphine after the neuromata which had developed in the amputated stump of his thumb had become so painful that he required constant pain-killers. Fleischl hated the way morphine dulled his mind, made several unsuccessful attempts to give it up, and was in the throes of the withdrawal sickness attending his latest attempt when Freud brought him the cocaine. According to Ernest Jones, "Fleischl clutched at the new drug 'like a drowning man' and within a few days was taking it continually."[26] However he "clutched" at it, cocaine made the withdrawal from morphine much more bearable.[27]

Fleischl's initial positive reaction to cocaine and his own success with it made Freud increasingly enthusiastic. He wrote to Martha that he took "very small doses of it regularly against depression and against indigestion, and with the most brilliant success. . . . If things go on in this way we need have no concern about being able to come together and stay in Vienna."[28] The euphoric quality of cocaine is readily discernible in this letter to Martha. Before this the chance of gaining a reputation that would assure him a thriving practice had seemed remote and no doubt contributed much to the depressions he suffered. But now, after taking cocaine, Freud is filled with high spirits and optimism. As Dr. J. Leonard Corning wrote in 1908, one of the more notable effects of cocaine is how "a sudden access of optimism causes enterprises that loomed impossible to take on an aspect of feasibility."[29]

Freud did something else common to drug takers—he passed it on: "He sent some to Martha 'to make her strong and give her cheeks a red color', he pressed it on his friends and colleagues both for themselves and their patients, and he gave it to his sister."[30] And he quickly began gathering together the literature on coca and cocaine for his own "song of praise to this magical substance."[31] Magical indeed. On April 21 he had not yet received his cocaine. By June 5 he had half-finished his song of praise, *Uber Coca,* and by June 10 he had completed it. Published the following month, it was the most complete account of cocaine yet to appear. He gave a detailed history of the coca plant, surveyed the current scientific literature, and reported the effects of cocaine on himself.

Uber Coca and the cocaine papers which followed are—excepting the last, *Craving For and Fear of Cocaine,* a reply to his critics—classic originals in a field which didn't receive its name until 1920.[32] That field, Psychopharmacology, is the study of drugs which modify thinking and behavior, and Freud's methodology has not been significantly improved upon. He carefully noted the size of the dose, its effect on his body and mind, the correlation between the two, and how the effects changed during the time of the drug's course of action. For those who may believe that Freud's results were suspect because he took the drug himself and thus was to some extent subjectively involved, I shall at this point only remark that not only is Freud's data not out of date, but that, with respect to cocaine's psychoactive properties, his data are far more accurate than anything you will find in the most authoritative current pharmacological texts.[33]

Getting back to *Uber Coca,* Freud writes: ". . . in doses of 0.05-0.10 gram [there is] exhilaration and lasting euphoria, which in no way differs from the normal euphoria of a healthy person. . . . One feels an increase of self-control and possesses more vitality and capacity for work . . . it is hard to believe that one is under the influence of any drug. . . . Long intensive mental or physical work is performed without any fatigue. . . . This result is enjoyed without any of the unpleasant aftereffects that follow exhilaration brought about by alcohol. . . . Absolutely no craving for the further use of cocaine appears after the first, or even repeated taking of the drug."[84] And Freud fully understood what few people do who obtain their information on psychoactive drugs from standard texts: that individual responses to such drugs vary greatly. He wrote: "I have had the opportunity of observing the effect of cocaine on quite a number of people; and on the basis of my findings I must stress, even more emphatically than before, the variation in individual reactions to cocaine. I found some individuals who showed signs of coca euphoria exactly like my own and others who experienced absolutely no effect from doses of 0.05-0.10 g. Yet others reacted to coca with symptoms of slight intoxication, marked by talkativeness and giddy behavior. On the other hand, an increased capacity for works seem to me to be a constant symptom."[85]

Freud enumerated seven likely therapeutic uses for cocaine: as a stimulant and, in that capacity, as a possible therapy for those suffering depression (The opiates were useful in calming hysterics, but until the advent of cocaine there was nothing available for the relief of depression.); for digestive disturbances; for the treatment of tuberculosis; for withdrawing alcohol and morphine addicts; for the alleviation of asthma; as an aphrodisiac; and as a local anesthetic.[36] Cocaine's anesthetic, stimulant, and aphrodisiac properties have been well established. Of the remainder of Freud's suggestions, some are doubtful, others are decidedly mistaken. Because of its anesthetic effects, oral doses of cocaine might very well relieve the pain of indigestion and, because it dampens appetite, it might very well eliminate one of the causes of indigestion—but there is no evidence to suggest it would help the more serious digestive disturbances. Nor has cocaine proved to be an effective treatment for tuberculosis. Its effectiveness has not been established in treating asthma, though it was for many years the basic ingredient of several patent medicine asthma cures.[37] And though cocaine had been much touted in America as a morphine cure since 1880, these reports and Freud's enthusiasm were somewhat premature. Cocaine undoubtedly did ease the pains of withdrawing from morphine insofar as it replaced languor and bodily distress with euphoria and feelings of energy, but the long-term benefits were less than impressive. In most cases the patients returned to morphine. Occasionally, they discovered they preferred a central nervous system *stimulant* to a central nervous system *depressant* and became heavy cocaine users. And, people being the ingenious creatures they are, a goodly number probably became the first of the speed-ballers, using morphine and cocaine together.[38]

Fleischl was one of those who found he preferred cocaine to morphine. Freud had shared his first gram of cocaine with him in the spring of 1884, and he had taken it in small doses similar to those taken by Freud. By January of 1885, however, Fleischl was up to a gram (15.4 grains) a day, a dosage he apparently continued through June 4—by which time he had developed cocaine poisoning with attendant psychotic reactions, seeing "white snakes creeping over his skin."[39] (Such a reaction is very similar to alcoholic delirium tremens.) This greatly disturbed Freud but it did not stop him from using and advocating cocaine. He also kept sending it to Martha, warning her to be moderate and to not acquire a habit.[40] Freud understood that cocaine offered no problems to moderate users. And though he characterized Fleischl's doses as "frightful," he was surely aware that the difference between his own daily intake and Fleischl's was *not* on the order described by his biographer Jones: "Fleischl was taking enormous doses of cocaine . . . a full gram a day—a hundred times the quantity Freud was accustomed to take."[41] But even if Freud had taken only one 0.05-0.10 gram dose per day he was ingesting one-twentieth to one-tenth of a gram, *not* one-hundredth of a gram, and his cocaine papers suggest that he usually took *more* than one dose per day. "If cocaine is used as a stimulant, it is best to administer it in small effective doses (0.05-0.10 gram), repeated so often that the effects of the doses overlap."[42] Since Freud primarily took cocaine as a stimulant, it is reasonable to assume that his daily intake was considerably in excess of a twentieth or a tenth of a gram. One can only estimate the number of doses he took in a day but he noted the marked effects of an oral dose lasted four to five hours.[43] This, with his admonition to overlap doses, makes it highly likely that he took at least two doses a day, and probable that he took three. All in all I should estimate Freud's intake of cocaine to be comparable to that of a moderate user today.[44]

As for Fleischl's "frightful" doses, most authorities consider it a proven fact that "repeated use of large doses of cocaine produces a characteristic paranoid psychosis in all or almost all users."[45] This is simply not true, whatever is meant by "large" doses. I must postpone full discussion to the last chapter, but right here it should be noted that Fleischl's gram a day—though a generous amount—is a great deal less than many cocaine users take over a period of years, and that he experienced psychosis only after several months of this constant daily usage. What neither Freud nor Fleischl knew was that cocaine in such amounts has a cumulative toxic effect.[46] Current habitual users understand this, which is why they periodically lay off cocaine when they begin to detect the signs of this accumulation.[47]

Between the publishing of *Uber Coca* in 1884 and his fifth and last paper on cocaine in 1887, Freud came under heavy attack for his advocacy of the drug. Fleischl's case was simply one of many bad reactions resulting from an overindulgence in cocaine. By 1887 most members of the European medical community were dead set against the use of cocaine except as a local anesthetic. The leading addiction specialist of the period accused Freud of unleashing the "third scourge of humanity" (after alcohol and morphine).[48] Freud's professional reputation was at stake, and to save it he abandoned the advocacy of cocaine. But he did not do so because he believed he was wrong and his critics right. In his final paper, *Craving For and Fear of Cocaine,* he argued heatedly, and correctly, that cocaine dependence was a rare occurrence and that so useful a drug should not be condemned simply because some people misused it. Such persons, he wrote, ". . . would abuse, and indeed did abuse, any stimulant offered them."[49]

It is generally thought that Freud gave up the personal use of cocaine in 1887, after the criticism he had received and the flood of reports of cocaine "addiction" had made its advocacy a professional liability— but there is definite proof that he used it at least in a therapeutic way (applied locally to "swellings in his nose") as late as 1895.[50] Whether he used it as a stimulant after 1887 cannot be determined by the available evidence, but however he used it there is no indication he ever experienced any difficulty with it. The canard printed in one recent popular book to the effect that Freud's excessive indulgence in cocaine resulted in three separate nose operations is without basis in fact.[51] So far as anyone knows, Freud never snorted cocaine—the applications to his nose were in the form of cocaine paste. He began by taking it orally, then switched to subcutaneous injections. His operations were for cancer of the palate and jaw, a disease he incurred as a result of smoking far too many cigars.[52]

Cocaine has long been, and continues to be, a highly valued stimulant, but no one other than the coca-chewing Indians of the Andes can use it as a stimulant without running the danger of being arrested. For outside its natural habitat, cocaine is considered an especially dangerous drug justifying the severest penalties. Its one legal use in most of the world is as a local anesthetic and, as with the isolation of cocaine from the coca leaf, there is considerable controversy

41

over who deserves the credit for having first recognized and demonstrated its value as a local anesthetic. Or, rather, there is controversy over which nineteenth-century European man of science deserves the honor—for there is indisputable anthropological evidence that the Indians used cocaine in surgical operations several hundred years before cocaine was known to the West.[53]

It seems likely that the Indians, understanding cocaine's anesthetic properties, used it in a variety of operations but the existing evidence points to only one kind—trepanning. This involves cutting out disks of bone from the skull, a dangerous operation in which many patients probably succumbed to the tender ministrations of the surgeon rather than to their injury or illness. Trepanning was employed to cure headaches and mental illness—the idea being that cutting out a portion of the skull would relieve the "pressure" causing these problems—as well as complex skull fractures. It might rightly be said that the Incas and their predecessors were as enamored of drastic remedies as are those current practitioners of psychosurgery who find the removal of part of the brain an appropriate remedy for certain mental health problems. But however inappropriate some of the trepanning operations may have been, they were at least relatively painless. After applying the cocaine-rich saliva from chewed coca leaves, the Indian surgeons were able to operate on a quiet, stationary object. Imagine the fatal slips of the knife had they been required to do their work on an unanesthetized, kicking and screaming patient.

Likewise, try to imagine undergoing an eye operation without benefit of anesthetic—which would have been your fate had you been so unfortunate as to require one prior to 1884. Western medicine had long since foregone trepanning, and limbs were not sawn off sans anesthetic well before Freud wrote his first monograph on cocaine. But there were surgical procedures for which general anesthetics such as ether were unsuitable. Chief among these were eye operations.[54] As Karl Koller, the man who first used cocaine in human eye surgery, wrote, "The immediate cause of my approaching the questions of local anesthesia was the unsuitability of general narcosis in eye operations—eye operations were . . . being done without any anesthetic whatever."[55] It must have been a nightmare: the terrible fear and pain of the patient, the surgeon attempting a delicate operation on a surface which could not be expected to remain still.

Given the great need for an effective local anesthetic, the great wonder is that it took so long for cocaine's anesthetic properties to be recognized. Or, more correctly, that it took so long for the scientists who were searching for a local anesthetic to make a simple, logical connection. Koller demonstrated cocaine's effectiveness in this regard in 1884, but it had been known since at least 1862 that the drug numbed the mucous membranes when applied locally. Indeed the anesthetizing effects of coca had been remarked upon by European writers for centuries. All who chewed coca observed that it made their lips and tongue numb.[56] And when cocaine was isolated from coca, it was quickly recognized that *this* was the ingredient which caused the numbing. Schroff read a paper before the Viennese Medical Society in 1862 in which he pointed out that cocaine numbed the tongue and dilated the pupils.[57] Six years later Thomas Moreno y Maiz published a paper in which, after describing his experiments, he suggested cocaine's usefulness as a local anesthetic.[58] Then in 1876 Charles Fauvel reported cocaine's anesthetizing effect on the mucous membranes.[59] And in 1879 von Anrep wrote an experimental paper describing, once again, the anesthetization of the mucous membranes and the dilation of the pupil by cocaine.[60] Von Anrep apparently failed to notice that the pupil also was desensitized as well as dilated or, if he did, to remark on it. (He may, in fact, have failed to appreciate the significance of his experiments altogether.)[61]

But if researchers such as von Anrep didn't appreciate the importance of their experiments, neither did the surgeons seeking a local anesthetic. Carl Koller, who had been obsessed with finding an anesthetic suitable for eye surgery, had, while studying at the University, read and underlined the following passage on cocaine. "Local effects: Injection under the skin as well as painting the mucous membranes, for example, the tongue—brings about the loss of feeling and pain. 15 minutes after painting it von Anrep was incapable of distinguishing sugar, salt and sour at the treated spot. Even the needle pricks could no longer be felt there, whereas the other unpainted side reacted normally. The loss of sensibility lasted between 25 and 100 minutes."[62]

Koller, first as a medical student and then as a doctor, could have no doubts that the surface of the eye was a mucous membrane; yet even after the publication of his friend Freud's first cocaine paper suggesting cocaine's usefulness as a local anesthetic, and despite his own reading in the literature on cocaine, he failed to grasp its possibilities for eye surgery. Not until in actual possession of cocaine—Freud had persuaded Koller to assist him in studying the physiological effects of cocaine—and then not until after another colleague had eaten some cocaine from *the point of a knife* and had remarked on its numbing effect, did Koller finally see the connection. He then immediately proceeded to the laboratory, applied cocaine to the cornea of a frog and found that he could prick the cornea with the point of a needle and elicit no response from the frog. He repeated the experiment on warm-blooded animals—dogs and rabbits, then on himself and a friend—and convinced himself he had at last discovered an effective local anesthetic. These experiments were conducted in early September, 1884, and Koller's paper and a practical demonstration of the experiment were given at the Heidelberg Ophthalmological Society on September 15, 1884.[63]

The honor of firmly establishing cocaine's effectiveness as a local anesthetic must go to Koller, but we are equally indebted to Freud for this discovery. Not only did he urge Koller to study the physiological effects of cocaine and suggest its usefulness as a local

44

anesthetic in his first paper, but *Uber Coca* also renewed the European medical community's interest in cocaine. This interest had been sporadically lively, but it never seemed to last very long. Many experiments were performed and after each new one interest lapsed. In England and on the Continent, cocaine was repeatedly dismissed as a drug of no practical value.[64] There were several reasons for this, some of which have already been mentioned. To begin with, the early manufacturers of cocaine produced a product which was neither uniform nor standardized—a state of affairs which probably accounts for the many contradictory and inconclusive results obtained in the experiments.[65] Then too, as Freud wrote, ". . . the current inflated price of the drug is an obstacle to any further investigations."[66] It is also possible that the psychotropic effects of cocaine (euphoria, endurance, mental clarity) were so striking when experienced that they overshadowed the simpler, anesthetic effect. Just why these striking effects, which had been commented on for centuries, should have been considered of no practical value is hard to understand, let alone explain.

Experiments on cocaine's local anesthetic properties were not confined to Europe. In the same year Koller did his experiments a young American surgeon was doing equally important work in this area. Before getting into that, however, it is worth noting that Koller had been taking cocaine during the months preceding his discovery. Freud had enlisted him for a series of tests to determine whether cocaine increased muscular strength. They would test themselves on a dynamometer; then take cocaine and repeat the tests. The cocaine improved their performances considerably.[67] And though there is no documentary evidence that Koller used cocaine apart from these and his own experiments, it is not easy to imagine he did not. He had a supply of cocaine, the drug was not considered dangerous, and he had been exposed to its euphoric and stimulating qualities. There was every reason to use it and none, except price, to discourage its use.

Fleischl had not yet developed his cocaine psychosis and his friend Freud was very enthusiastic about the drug. I think it reasonable, therefore, to suppose that Koller occasionally dipped into the coke bottle for reasons other than the work at hand. I make this conjecture because I find it striking that three months after first using cocaine, Koller saw what for several years he had been unable to see: the connection between cocaine's numbing effect on the mucous membranes and its application as a local anesthetic in eye surgery. The cerebral stimulation afforded by cocaine may have had nothing to do with his belated insight, but the possibility should not be discounted.

Meanwhile in America, William Stewart Halsted, the man who has been called the father of modern surgery, was attempting to inject cocaine into a nerve center in the hope of producing anesthesia in the area served by the nerves. At about the same time Koller was demonstrating his new technique, Halsted succeeded in performing the first "nerve block."[68] He wrote several articles describing his technique in 1885 and then wasn't heard from for a year. What had happened was that Halsted, like all conscientious researchers, had used himself as a guinea pig and had acquired a good-sized cocaine habit. It isn't clear how long he was a heavy user, but circumstantial evidence makes it likely that he used almost two grams a day for about a year.[69] Just what was his mental state at the end of this period is not clear either, but Sir Wilder Penfield, himself a famous surgeon, later wrote that Halsted's chronic indulgence in cocaine resulted in a "confused and unworthy period of medical practice."[70] At any rate, Dr. William H. Welch, one of the founders of Johns Hopkins Medical School and Halsted's closest friend, decided that Halsted had to be weaned from cocaine. To effect this he hired a schooner and with three crewmen took Halsted on a slow trip to the Windward Islands and back—the idea being that once on the open sea there would be no way for Halsted to procure cocaine. There wasn't and, according to Penfield, when they returned the once "brilliant and gay extrovert seemed brilliant and gay no longer."[71]

Apparently Halsted preferred being brilliant and gay to being dull and introverted because he immediately got back into cocaine. He subsequently spent several months at Butler Hospital in Providence, Rhode Island, trying once again to cure his desire for cocaine. He didn't succeed, took it up again, then entered Butler a second time. According to his biographers, this second trip was a great success. Halsted, with great strength of will, etc., etc., cast out the demon cocaine and went on to become a "great and successful surgeon." He certainly did become a very famous surgeon, but he needed more than strength of will to give up his cocaine. What in fact happened was that Halsted "cured" his cocaine habit with morphine, and was a morphine addict from 1886 until his death in 1922 at the age of 70. During this long period of addiction, Halsted developed an operating technique which stressed not only minimum damage to tissues but also the natural process of repair to damaged tissues. And he introduced, as part of his concept of preventing the introduction of germs into a wound, the use of rubber gloves. For these and other major innovations he has been rightly called the "father of modern surgery." Addiction to morphine didn't impair his progress in the least. He was active and in good health to the very end.[72]

Fleischl, a brilliant physician and friend of Freud, took cocaine to wean himself from morphine; Halsted, the brilliant surgeon, took morphine to wean himself from cocaine. Both were successful insofar as they got off the drug they wanted to get off, but Fleischl suffered toxic reactions from cocaine whereas Halsted lived a happy active life addicted to morphine. Does this mean that cocaine is "bad" and morphine "good?" No, it only means that cocaine wasn't good for Fleischl and morphine wasn't bad for Halsted. The positive and negative effects of cocaine will be discussed at length later on, but before going further into the story of cocaine it seems worthwhile to say something about the manner in which we use moral terms to characterize drugs.

For example, penicillin is universally considered a "good" drug, heroin a "bad" one. If you stop to think about it, this is a very odd way to talk about drugs. "Good" and "bad" are moral terms, not scientific terms. When doctors and pharmacologists say a drug is "good" they usually mean that it is effective for its purpose. Yet both penicillin and heroin are highly effective for their purposes—the one as an antibiotic, the other as a pain-killer—and one is called "good," the other "bad." Of course there is a reason for the distinction. Drugs have a whole range of effects, not all of which are directly connected to the purposes for which they are prescribed. That is, drugs have side effects.

Among other things penicillin destroys the intestinal bacteria which synthesizes vitamin B and thus destroys our most important source of the vitamin. And anyone who regularly uses heroin over a sufficient length of time will become addicted to it. In this sense both penicillin and heroin are "bad" drugs. A consensus has developed, however, that on balance the positive effects of penicillin far outweigh the negative, whereas the negative effects of heroin far outweigh the positive. Thus penicillin is "good" and heroin "bad." But penicillin is certainly not good for those allergic to it— it can and has killed them; and heroin is not bad for those who need a pain-killer stronger than morphine.

No drug in the pharmacopoeia, whether licit or illicit, is good or bad in and of itself. It can be properly so characterized only in relation to individual cases. Or, Freud fared well on cocaine, Fleischl badly. Our laws may declare a drug "bad" and its possession for unauthorized use a crime, but this says nothing about the drug itself; it only reflects the official attitude towards it. And it can be safely said that none of the long list of drugs we use only on the pain of possible imprisonment became illicit drugs as a result

48

of careful, objective testing. As we shall see, the most important factors in the prohibiting of certain drugs have been racism, politics, greed, and ignorance.

3

The Great Boom

The publicity given to Koller's demonstration of
cocaine's value as a local anesthetic made the drug
known to virtually every doctor in Europe and America
and to most of the educated public as well. Newspapers and magazines heralded the new wonder drug,
and medical journals carried accounts which came close
to advocating an unlimited intake of cocaine.[1] Physicians of great repute heartily endorsed it for purposes
which could be called medical only by stretching the
meaning of the term beyond reasonable bounds. In
America, the former surgeon general of the Army,
William Hammond, proudly informed the public he
used cocaine as a tonic and stimulant on a daily basis,
found it constantly refreshing, and never suffered any
subsequent depression.[2] In England, the 78-year-old
president of the British Medical Association, Sir Robert
Christison, wrote an enthusiastic report describing how
under the stimulus of cocaine he had been able to
take fifteen-mile hikes and climb mountains with

"youthful vigor" and no feelings of fatigue.[3] And in Germany, of course, there was Freud writing songs of praise to cocaine, conducting careful research, passing it on to his friends, and stimulating other researchers into further investigations of the drug.

Since people are usually more than willing to heed the advice of doctors who recommend what makes them feel good, the enthusiasm of the physicians would have been enough to make cocaine a commodity much sought after by the general public. But as modern advertising has so excruciatingly demonstrated, the more frequently a product is mentioned the better its chances of acceptance. Whatever his intentions, Sir Arthur Conan Doyle most certainly increased the recognition rating of cocaine when he made Sherlock Holmes a user. More accurately, perhaps, he *reinforced* an awareness already present in his readers. For no author with so sure a grasp of popular taste would provide his leading character with a habit so unfamiliar to his readers that they could have no idea of its implications. Conan Doyle would not, for example, have made Holmes a devotee of Buddhist meditations. He was well aware that few of his readers knew anything about meditation, just as he knew that most of them had heard something about cocaine. It isn't likely they knew much. If Conan Doyle's initial fund of knowledge on the subject is any indication, it is probable they knew little more than that cocaine was a drug with striking effects.

The first mention of cocaine in the Holmes stories comes in "A Scandal in Bohemia," written in 1886, one year after an eminent critic of Freud had condemned cocaine as an addictive drug worse than morphine.[4] This linking of the two very different drugs apparently led some people, Conan Doyle among them, to incorrectly assume that the effects of cocaine and morphine were similar—an assumption perhaps strengthened by the fact that morphine had been initially considered a cure for opium addiction, as at this juncture cocaine was being touted as a cure for morphine addiction. Morphine was like opium, only

51

more so; and it might have seemed logical to believe that cocaine was like morphine, only more so. However this may be, Conan Doyle, who was trained as a doctor, did not in 1886 know the difference between the two. He has Holmes "alternating from week to week between cocaine and ambition, the drowsiness of the drug and the fierce energy of his own keen nature," and goes on to relate how Holmes "had risen out of his drug-created dreams, and was hot upon the scent of some new problem."[5] Now this sounds very like opium or morphine, not at all like cocaine. The "drowsiness of the drug" and "drug-created dreams" aptly describe the effects of the opiates but are totally inappropriate when applied to cocaine; to say nothing of the fact that cocaine is an ambition-inducing drug, not, as Conan Doyle implies, the opposite. (Later writers of popular detective fiction were equally confused. For example Sax Rohmer never managed to get the distinction between cocaine and the opiates straight in any of his Fu-Manchu novels; and Dashiell Hammett in *The Dain Curse,* a novel in which drugs play an important role, had the same problem.)

By 1888, however, he had learned a good deal about cocaine. Consider the following extracts from the "The Sign of the Four," all of which occur after Watson has described Holmes "sinewy forearms and wrist, all dotted and scarred with innumerable puncture-marks," and has related how he has watched Holmes shooting cocaine three times a day for many months:

"Which is it to-day?" I asked. "Morphine or cocaine?"

"It is cocaine," he said. ". . . Would you care to try it?"

"No indeed," I answered, brusquely. "My constitution has not got over the Afghan campaign yet. I cannot afford to throw any extra strain upon it."

He smiled at my vehemence. "Perhaps you are right, Watson," he said.

"I suppose that its influence is physically a bad one. I find it, however, so transcendingly stimulating and clarifying to the mind that its secondary action is a matter of small moment."

"But consider!" I said, earnestly. "Count the cost! . . . You know, too, what a black reaction comes upon you. . . ."

A bit later, Holmes further expands on his reasons for taking cocaine:

"My mind," he said, "rebels at stagnation. Give me problems, give me work . . . and I am in my own proper atmosphere, I can dispense then with artificial stimulants. But I abhor the dull routine of existence. I crave for mental exaltation."

Though not relevant to the issue, the ending of "The Sign of the Four" has such a nice touch that I shall give it for the benefit of those who do not have a copy of the story. After the episodes just described a client appears and, to Watson's great relief, Holmes sets aside the cocaine. He solves the problem with his usual sagacity and energy, and Watson, as they are discussing the case, comments:

"The division seems rather unfair. . . . You have done all the work in this business. I get a wife out of it, Jones gets the credit, pray, what remains for you?"

"For me," said Sherlock Holmes, "there still remains the cocaine bottle."

And he stretched his long white hand up for it.

Taking into account the marked improvement in Conan Doyle's knowledge of the effects of cocaine which took place in the two years between "A Scandal in Bohemia" and "The Sign of the Four," the level of ignorance from which he started, and the lack of understanding exhibited by trained medical researchers who had never taken cocaine, it seems possible that Conan Doyle relied upon something more than second-hand facts. Indeed when one reads the 1891 story,

"The Final Problem" it is clear that Conan Doyle had also learned much about the effects of long-term overindulgence in cocaine. The master detective, paler and thinner than ever, is exhibiting classic paranoid fantasies about the archcriminal Moriarty:

"For years I have been continually convinced of some power behind the malefactor, some deep organizing power which forever stands in the way of the law and throws its shield over the wrongdoer."

He is also certain that Moriarty is trying to kill him, but for neither case does he offer any evidence beyond his own deductive certainty. He takes commonplace events as "evidence" to support his darkest doubts. When the Alpine guide says that a fall of rocks is to be expected at this time and place, Holmes makes no verbal comment, but smiles "with the air of a man who sees the fulfillment of that which he had expected." In short, the picture painted by the good Dr. Watson of Holmes's appearance and exceedingly suspicious turn of mind is an accurate portrait of the behavior and appearance of someone suffering toxic and psychotic reactions to cocaine.

To deduce from the evidence in the Holmes stories that Conan Doyle did himself undergo these cocaine rites of passage is admittedly a bit presumptuous, based as the deduction is on evidence just a trifle more substantial than that which Holmes customarily employed to reach his paranoid conclusions respecting Moriarty and the power behind him. So take it as you will.

Sir Arthur wasn't the only English man of letters to make use of cocaine's new notoriety. Dr. Myron Schultz has advanced the hypothesis that the powerful drug taken by Dr. Jekyll which transformed him into the evil Mr. Hyde was none other than cocaine. Moreover, Dr. Schultz makes a strong case for believing that Stevenson wrote his popular novel in the Autumn of 1885 under the influence of cocaine. The medical evidence he offers supports this conclusion, but his literary evidence is much stronger: in *three days* the sickly Robert Louis Stevenson wrote a first draft, burnt it, and then in another three days composed a second and finished version, a total of 60,000 words.[6] The most fluent hacks usually take at least three weeks to pound out a third-rate detective novel of that length. And they do their writing on electric typewriters.

The publicity given cocaine was better than money could buy: unsolicited testimonials from eminent authorities, continual coverage by the media of the day, and enough controversy to ensure its being kept in the public consciousness. Useless products have been successfully promoted with none of these advantages. Given a product as saleable as cocaine, great success was inevitable. The public bought it if not in every conceivable form, in as wide a variety of concoctions as any drug had hitherto or has since been packaged. Cocaine was sold in wine, in soda pop, in tea, in cigarettes, in chewing gum, in nose sprays and nose powders, and in any number of patent medicines. And it was sold simply as 100 per cent pure cocaine from the best of laboratories, available at the local drugstore, no prescription necessary, and no signature required.

And though Yankee entrepreneurs outdid Europe in the quantity and variety of cocaine items they manufactured and sold, it was a Corsican residing in Paris who led the great cocaine explosion by demonstrating how profitable it could be. Angelo Mariani was born in Bastia, a major city of Corsica, of a family of physicians and chemists.[7] His adult life was devoted to studying coca and finding a way to capture its essence in an appetizing and marketable form. An earlier Corsican more vividly captured the world's imagination but his conquests were neither as extensive nor as long-lived as Mariani's, whose coca products were sold all over the Western Hemisphere for more than thirty years. Napoleon led his armies to glory, but Mariani performed a more useful service— he gave his followers pleasure and a sense of well-being. Pope Leo XIII, who for many years was "supported in his ascetic retirement by a preparation of Mariani's coca," expressed his ecclesiastical approval by presenting Mariani with a gold medal and citing him as a benefactor of humanity.[8] The president of the Académie des Beaux Arts did likewise.[9] The composers Gounod, Fauré, and Massenet extolled him in song.[10] The most distinguished physicians of the era offered glowing testimonials:

Dr. Charles Fauvel of Paris, an early and noted cocaine researcher—

"Thanks to Mariani wine I have been able to restore the voice of many lyric artists who would have been unable without this potent agent to give their performances."[11]

Dr. J. Leonard Corning of New York, who first suggested the use of cocaine for spinal anesthesia—

"Of Vin Mariani I need hardly speak as the medical profession is already aware of its virtues. Of all the tonic preparations ever introduced to the notice of the profession, this is undoubtedly the most potent for good in the treatment of exhaustive and irritative conditions of the central nervous system."[12]

Endorsements from eminent personages were so numerous that Mariani, an exceedingly shrewd public relations man, compiled and published them in a handsome biographical encyclopedia. Each well-known endorser of Vin Mariani was accorded an entry which included an outline of his career, an etched portrait, and suitable quotations from his testimonials. The encyclopedia, a deluxe production with the best of paper, typography, and binding, ran to several large volumes and quickly became a collector's item.[13] Queen Victoria, on receiving a set, wrote Mariani that she considered the volumes the "finest specimens in her collection."[14]

(The volumes are rare and I have not been able to

locate a set. The endorsers of Mariani products I have mentioned were garnered from secondary sources. And though it would be nice to list all of Vin Mariani's celebrated enthusiasts, it would probably be easier to list the late nineteenth- and early twentieth-century notables who were *not* enthusiasts. From what I can gather, Vin Mariani was as popular in its day as Coca-Cola is now.)

Mariani introduced his wine to the public in either 1863 or 1865.[15] In 1872 he published a short article, "La Coca du Pérou," in a small therapeutic journal.[16] This effort was followed in 1878 by the first two volumes on the history and therapeutic applications of coca; the second volume appeared in 1888, and a translation was published in New York in 1896.[17]

All of Mariani's coca products—and, in addition to Vin Mariani, there were Mariani's elixir, Mariani's lozenges, Mariani's pastilles, and Mariani's tea—contained generous portions of coca's chief alkaloid, cocaine. Their popularity was so great that Mariani became the largest importer of coca leaves in Europe, surpassing even those pharmaceutical houses which manufactured great quantities of cocaine.[18]

According to the most knowledgeable historian of coca, Mariani knew more about the chemistry of coca than anyone in Europe or America.[19] And judging by the success of his business ventures, he had few peers as an entrepreneur. But he was more than an able chemist with finely honed business instincts—he was something of an alchemist who apparently believed that in coca he had found the philosopher's stone, the very elixir of life.[20] He was also, as you might expect, a lover of coca: ". . . Coca is the hobby of Mariani. It is his recreation, his relaxation and constant source of pleasure, wholly removed from sordid commercial interests. At Neuilly, on the Seine, Paris, France, where his laboratory is located, his study is tastefully arranged with rich tapestries and carvings, in which the . . . Coca leaf and flower are so artistically used as the motif of decoration that they are not obtrusive but

57

must be pointed out in order to be recognized."[21] Or, loving your work never hurts.

(This is pure speculation, but I cannot help thinking that a design so subtle that it had to "be pointed out in order to be recognized" was neither accidental nor simply a matter of taste. Mariani knew a lot about coca and cocaine and surely was aware that most novices didn't recognize the specific effects of the drug until they were pointed out to them. I like to think, then, that the subtlety of his coca motifs was a metaphor for the drug experience itself; and perhaps even a reminder that coca and cocaine were best when used in moderation.)

As great as was Mariani's success in Europe, it seems it was even greater in America.[22] I have not been able to ascertain the volume of his business either here or abroad, but it was large enough to make him a very rich man. And, more significantly, large enough to spawn a host of imitators. For though cocaine, which had first achieved popularity in America as a cure for opiate addiction—did your mother, father, sister, brother, son, or daughter have a problem with opium or morphine? cocaine can save them from a fate worse than death—was by the 1890s no longer being heavily pushed for this purpose, a drug which made so many people feel so good clearly had its virtues and the success of Vin Mariani had made its commercial potential obvious. The doctors and the patent medicine industry soon found any number of uses for it, and cocaine quickly became popular as a general tonic and stimulant, a cure for the common cold, and a remedy for asthma, hay fever, and sinusitis.

With the exception of its demonstrated ability to pep people up, cocaine was not a specific remedy for any of these ailments—though some of its properties might have led doctors and laymen to suppose it was. Cocaine does, after all, dry up the mucous membranes and enough of it will drain the sinus cavities as well. Hay fever and sinus sufferers, therefore, could easily believe their conditions relieved. As indeed they were, temporarily. Ditto the common cold. And cocaine's numbing effect on the nose, throat, and lungs might well afford temporary relief to asthma victims. Providing then as it did euphoria and energy as well as temporary relief of very common ailments, cocaine could hardly fail to reach an enthusiastic public. Who wouldn't buy and take a medicine with such pleasant side effects?

Those who now use cocaine feel equally enthusiastic about it, but they don't have easy access to it. They not only must pay very high prices but they must search out a supplier. The situation was very different in nineteenth-century America, a place and time which has been called a "dope fiend's paradise."[23] Any drug one might wish to use was both cheap and legal, and as easy to get as a pack of cigarettes. Like opium and morphine, cocaine could be obtained from your doctor; over the counter from the druggist; at the grocery or general store; in the mail from any of numerous mail-order houses who stocked and sold drugs; and, finally, if you were a typical citizen of the times and didn't fancy yourself a "drug-user," you could simply buy one of the many patent medicines which contained cocaine. (Along these lines it should be noted that, since there were no laws requiring the manufacturer to list the ingredients, and many patent medicine and proprietary remedy makers didn't list them, many cocaine users probably had no idea they were taking cocaine, or opium, morphine, and a number of other powerful drugs.)[24]

Probably the first of Mariani's American imitators was John Styth Pemberton of Atlanta, Georgia, the proprietor of Triplex Liver Pills and Globe of Flower Cough Syrup, who in 1885 introduced a new product to his line: French Wine Coca - Ideal Nerve and Tonic Stimulant. Pemberton's wine was a frank takeoff on Mariani's but connoisseurs of the time pronounced Mariani's product a noticeably superior concoction.[25] Undaunted, in 1886 Pemberton introduced a syrup containing cocaine and caffeine to be used as the basis of a "soft" drink. The syrup, Coca-Cola, was advertised as a "remarkable therapeutic agent" and a "sovereign remedy."[26] It continued as a cocaine-based drink until 1903, when the pressure applied by Southerners who feared blacks' getting cocaine in any form and by those seeking passage of a pure food and drug act led the manufacturer to omit cocaine.[27]

Another Mariani competitor, Metcalf's Coca Wine, claimed to be capable of alleviating or curing, among other things, phthisis, typhus, scurvy, gastralgia, anemia, enteralgia, the opium habit, alcoholism, and indigestion. Most of these claims had no basis in fact and one must doubt that the average user of Metcalf's Coca Wine and similar products fully believed they were such wonder-working cure-alls. Thousands of patent medicines and tonics were available at the time, and hardly any of them exhibited any shyness in claiming power over countless disabilities and indispositions. There wasn't an affliction known to man for which some enterprising hustler didn't have a "cure" or "relief." From tuberculosis to the common cold, from menstrual cramps to impotency, from the pains of addiction to the misery of listlessness, and for anything else imaginable, a specific product was available. Indeed as in the case of Metcalf's, almost all of the proprietary nostrums were advertised as fit remedies for a number of ailments, real or imaginary. That average consumers could have been taken in by such extravagant claims seems unlikely to me. What *does* seem likely is that these claims afforded them a convenient rationale for taking the drug of their choice. Those who did not like to admit to themselves or to others that they were regular users of cocaine, opium, or alcohol—facts which could hardly be concealed if they drank openly in a public saloon or bought their cocaine and opium from the neighborhood druggist—had only to buy the appropriate patent medicine. And since few of us are so gloriously healthy that we never suffer from even minor indispositions, almost everyone had an excuse for using something. Just what proportion of the population did resort to these nostrums cannot be accurately estimated, but given the tremendous size of the patent medicine industry there is no question that the proportion was very large.[28]

The entrepreneurs who boldly stated their product could relieve or cure the list of troubles listed on the label always made sure that what its chief ingredient *really* could do received prominent mention. Metcalf's Coca Wine (A Pleasant Tonic and Invigorator) provides a beautiful example. After listing the specific ailments mentioned earlier and declaring the user could find relief by drinking one-half to one glass three times a day, the main body of the label gave a more truthful and more appealing story:

> "Coca leaves have been used by the native Indians of South America from the earliest times for every malady from headache to neuralgia; and while chewing it, they pass whole days in travelling or working without food, eating heartily in the evening, without inconvenience, and passing the night in refreshing slumber.
>
> "Public Speakers, Singers, and Actors have found Wine of Coca (Metcalf's) to be a valuable tonic to the vocal chords.
>
> "Athletes, Pedestrians, and Base Ball Players have found by practical experience that a steady course of coca taken both before and after any trial of strength or endurance will impart energy to every movement, and prevent fatigue.
>
> "Elderly people have found it a reliable aphrodisiac superior to any other drug."[29]

As was the case with many cocaine products, Metcalf's wine failed to mention how much of the drug was in each bottle. There is no way of telling, therefore, how much was consumed by the user who followed the instructions on the label. But analyses made of various popular nostrums of the period make it clear that the typical manufacturer did not stint on the active ingredients. Dr Tucker's Specific "For the Perfect Relief And Cure of Asthma, Hay Fever AND

Catarrh," for example, was found to contain seven grains of cocaine (almost one-half gram) to the ounce.[30] And Coca-Bola, "a chewing paste which acts as a powerful tonic to the muscular and nervous system, relieving fatigue and exhaustion, and enabling the user to perform additional mental and physical labor without evil after-effects," contained almost three-quarters of a gram per ounce.[31] Dr. C. L. Mitchell, the proprietor of Coca-Bola, advised his customers to take it at "intervals as needed throughout the day" and for the "full effect . . . to use several squares."[32] Given the amount of cocaine in his little item, Dr. Mitchell was wrong in assuring people there could be no evil after-effects, just as he was wrong in claiming that "as a remedy and substitute for TOBACCO, ALCOHOL, and OPIUM, in the treatment of those habits, it is invaluable."[33] He was correct, however, in stating that Coca-Bola was a powerful stimulant. A cheap one too: Coca-Bola sold for 50 cents a box (55 cents by mail).[34]

Dr. Tucker's Specific and Dr. Mitchell's Coca-Bola contained generous amounts of cocaine, but they were short-weighting the customer in comparison to some of the other popular nostrums. AZ-MA-SYDE, an asthma "cure" produced by the Asthma Remedy and Manufacturing Co. of Cornelia, Georgia, contained some four and one-half grams of cocaine to the fluid ounce.[35] Ryno's Hay Fever-n-Catarrh Remedy, "manufactured" by E. H. Ryno, Wayland, Michigan, was discovered to be 99.95 percent pure cocaine.[36]

And then there was Nyal's Compound Extract of Damiana, which though when compared to AZ-MA-SYDE and Ryno's was relatively mild—with "only" one gram of cocaine per fluid ounce—did make a claim which assured its success with all those who worried about their potency: "Damiana is used as an aphrodisiac and for the restoration of virility in debility of the reproductive organs of both sexes."[37] And I can't refrain from mentioning Paine's Celery Compound, "A Nerve Tonic and Alternative Medicine, which can justly be called one of the Great Things in the line of Aids to Health and Happiness."[38] Paine's consisted of cocaine and alcohol, and though it is not clear what medicine it was an alternative to, the *joie de vivre* of the promotional line makes it reasonably clear that either Paine or his copywriter (or both) were satisfied users of the alternative medicine.

What has just been given is but a sampling of the cocaine products available in the late nineteenth and early twentieth centuries. There were many, many more—and they were not confined to tonics and alleged remedies for specific ailments. Coca-Cola was the most famous of the soft drinks which contained cocaine and is the lone survivor, but it once had numerous competitors. In *Nostrums and Quackery,* a report issued by the American Medical Association, there appears the following list of "soft" drinks containing cocaine: Kos-Kola, Kola-Ade, Koca-Nola, Cafe-Coca Compound, Pilsbury's Coke Extract, Celery Cola, Coke Extract, Dr. Don's Kola, Vani-Kola Compound Syrup, Rococola, and Wiseola.[39] Allowing a dozen "soft" drinks laced with cocaine within easy reach of the kiddies would, in this day and age, bring down a president far faster than any flagrant abuse of the Constitution; but this list names only a few that were available, those few whose labels failed to mention cocaine after the Pure Food and Drug Act of 1906 had outlawed such omissions and which had judgments served on them for violating the Act. Koca-Nola was the worst offender. The others simply omitted to list cocaine on their label, but Koca-Nola had the temerity to proclaim itself the "Delicious Dopeless Koca-Nola" at a time when it contained as much cocaine as any of them.[40] To be absolutely fair, it's quite possible that the makers of Koca-Nola were not trying to fool the public, but rather were hoping to fool the authorities. For by 1910 and for reasons which shall be explained in the next chapter, many states had enacted anticocaine laws; the public, moreover, had long been aware that such drinks contained cocaine. Indeed during the seventeen years Coca-Cola contained cocaine, the drink and the drug became so closely identified that "dope," as in "let's have a dope" became the established, common term for Coca-Cola. So well established that it remained in ordinary use right through the 1930s, long after cocaine had disappeared from Coca-Cola.[41]

The hay fever, asthma, and common cold remedies, together with the tonics and soft drinks, undoubtedly accounted for most of the cocaine consumed in America during the nineteenth and early twentieth centuries. In 1905 a drug journal listed the names of over 28,000 patent medicines then being marketed; and in 1906 it was estimated that some 50,000 were being sold.[42] No one knows how many of these contained cocaine, but between 1904 and 1906 the importation of coca leaves increased dramatically. Treasury department figures for 1904 show that 3,625 pounds of cocaine and 53,000 pounds of coca leaves (enough to yield 500 pounds of cocaine) were imported; and in 1905, when a 25 per cent duty on refined cocaine had made it economically advantageous to refine cocaine here rather than import it, 1,560 pounds of cocaine and 300,000 pounds of coca leaves (enough to yield approximately 2,500 pounds of cocaine) were brought in. The cocaine yield in both years was roughly the same—4,125 pounds as opposed to 4,060 pounds—but in 1906 some 2,600,000 pounds of coca leaves (enough to make approximately 21,000 pounds of cocaine) reached America.[43] A rough idea of how much cocaine this represents may be gained by considering that (a) with cocaine the choicest, most "in" drug on the market today, federal agents believe that it is being smuggled into the United States at a rate of 22,000 pounds a year;[44] (b) the current population is in excess of 210,000,000; and (c) the population in 1906 was less than 90,000,000. Accepting the federal estimate, one could say Americans consumed as much coke in 1906 as they did in 1974, and there were less than half as many of them to do it. But federal estimates of the drug traffic are notoriously inaccurate and probably twice that much coke is now coming in. So we probably used about as much coke in 1906 as we do in 1974—which is a lot, as we shall later see.

From another perspective one could say they were using no more cocaine when it was legal than we are now when it is illegal. This fact radically undermines the prime argument of the drug prohibitionists—who stoutly maintain that whatever may be wrong with the drug laws, they at least cut down the use of "dangerous" drugs and that to legalize such drugs would result in such an increase in use that the nation would be ruined.

However the rate of cocaine use in the early 1900s compares with the present, cocaine was so common that one 1903 report cited a drugstore in Philadelphia where "regular customers can enter and get cocaine without any formality. . . . Holding up one finger means the party wants a 'five-cent powder'; two fingers, ten cents worth; three, fifteen cents, and so on, the mere holding up of the fingers . . . being enough!"[45] Or something like the way a clerk, on seeing a regular customer walk in, picks out the cigars he always buys and has them ready and waiting. And it was as cheap as it was common. An ounce of pure cocaine cost approximately $2.50 in 1906 in New York.[46] (Today in New York an 85 to 90 per cent pure ounce goes for about $2000.00. Prohibition does do *one* thing, it makes dealing illicit drugs a very profitable enterprise.)

The year 1906 marked the beginning of the end for the free and easy distribution of cocaine. Spurred by Samuel Hopkins Adams's exposé of the patent medicine industry and Upton Sinclair's novel, *The Jungle,* which in stomach-turning detail revealed the practices of the meat-packing industry, Congress at last passed the Pure Food and Drug Act.[47] And though the Act required only that manufacturers list ingredients on their labels and did not prohibit any specific ingredients, it soon eliminated the use of cocaine in patent medicines and other proprietary products. By 1912 almost all of the states had prohibited the sale of cocaine except by prescription,[48] and the great selling point of the patent medicines had been that they allowed the buyers to bypass the doctors and use whatever medication appealed to them. A drug, therefore, that had to be prescribed by a physician was no longer commercially viable for the medicine industry.

But neither the Pure Food and Drug Act of 1906, nor the various state anticocaine laws enacted prior to 1914 reduced the consumption of cocaine in America. Nor did the passage of the Harrison Act of 1914 (the first national antidrug law), which brought the power of the federal government to bear on anyone dispensing cocaine without a doctor's prescription, reduce consumption. On the contrary, where in 1906 some 21,000 pounds of cocaine were floating around the country, by 1919 the amount of legally distributed cocaine had risen to 26,000 pounds—to say nothing of all the cocaine distributed by the brisk illicit traffic which had developed over the previous several years.[49]

It is interesting to note that although the Pure Food and Drug Act and the subsequent laws broadening its scope greatly reduced the number of patent and proprietary medicine makers, and effectively stopped them from using cocaine, the opiates, and many other drugs in their over-the-counter preparations, the proprietary medicine business is bigger than ever. At the turn of the century its combined annual sales were in the millions, they are now in the billions.[50] The Proprietary Association, which in the past lobbied strenuously to defeat the Pure Food and Drug Act and other restrictive legislation, has learned over the years that it is profitable to comply with the law. As its president assured the downcast members back in 1906, "People will generally reason . . . that preparations which come up to the requirements of a congressional enactment must be all right, or, certainly, that they are not harmful or dangerous."[51] But aspirin, for example, can be, and frequently is, very harmful.

The notion that drugs controlled by federal statutes "must be all right" applies with even greater force

66

to the prescription drugs made by the members of the Pharmaceutical Manufacturers' Association. After all, what can be bad about what a doctor prescribes? But the laws simply give the manufacturers a legal monopoly, they don't, for example, make legal amphetamines any safer than black market amphetamines. Indeed most of the black market amphetamines are made by the same people who produce the legal stuff. The "ethical" drug industry produces billions of doses of amphetamines and barbiturates each year, and a significant part of the production is diverted to the illicit market in one way or another.[52]

As with the illicit dealer, the drug laws protect the legal seller's market. They permit the manufacturer to promote his goodies with a freedom that passes all sensible bounds. In 1973, "Twenty major drug concerns gave doctors more than two billion free samples of drugs. . ."[53] These same twenty companies sent "reminder gifts" valued at more than $14 millions to doctors, nurses, and other health professionals.[54] There is nothing like having the law on your side if you are a drug dealer.

No one should think that the drug companies now produce amphetamines instead of cocaine because amphetamines are *safer* than cocaine: As we shall later see, the effects of the amphetamines are analogous to those of cocaine, but they are both more striking and more potentially dangerous. They make amphetamines because they can be legally sold to a far wider market than cocaine. Indeed America's drug manufacturers have always made and sold whatever was most profitable. When it was legal, they had no scruples in flooding the country with opium, morphine, and heroin and cocaine products. The Parke, Davis Company, for example, was once a most enthusiastic promoter of cocaine; they sold it in flake crystals, tablets, solutions for injection, ointments, and nasal sprays. They even marketed coca-leaf cigarettes and cigars.[55] When this was no longer legally permissible, they and their brethren didn't go out of business, they simply switched to other psychoactive drugs—

like the amphetamines which, though they didn't come on the market until the 1930s, have certainly proved to be more profitable than cocaine.

4

The Making of An "Especially Dangerous Drug"

Though few people outside the medical community had even heard of cocaine prior to 1880, it was already being widely used by 1885, and its use grew steadily over the next twenty years. First pushed to popularity by the lavish praise of the physicians, and then by the blatant advertising of the patent medicine industry, cocaine seemed the ideal drug for the industrious Americans. But before the end of the first decade of the twentieth century, the wondrous product which was to enable the citizenry to "face their second century of independence with the conveniently vigorous effects of a substance which 'never depresses,' has 'no re-coil,' and eliminates fatigue"[1] had been transformed into an especially dangerous drug, much as Dr. Jekyll had been transformed into Mr. Hyde.

Cocaine hadn't changed, opinions about its effects had. The energetic New Yorker who could snort all the coke he wanted in 1906, needed a doctor's prescription in 1907. He probably hadn't changed either, but according to the new law he was a sick man.

Before describing how this came about, it is worth trying to understand the more general question of why some drugs are accepted by the dominant culture of society and others rejected. This does not happen, as some might imagine, because careful tests have revealed that Drug A causes serious problems, Drug B doesn't, and therefore A is banned and B permitted. If this were the case, alcohol would be a black market drug and cocaine sold over the counter in drug stores.[2] Since this isn't the case, something more must be involved, a lot more in fact than I can possibly describe here. What I can do is give my interpretation of the facts; or, put another way, I can tell you how *I* see the situation.

To begin with, if there is any general rule on this question it is that the longer a drug is used in a society, the more likely it is to be either tolerated, or accepted, by those who wield power in the society. A corollary to this rule is that the more the established elite of a society use a drug, the more likely it is to be accepted by the society at large. For example, the number of people who smoke marijuana increases each year and each year a larger proportion of the business and professional classes smokes. Marijuana has become firmly entrenched in the culture. Which is why a presidential commission has stated that criminal sanctions against the drug serve no useful purpose,[3] at least one state has abandoned such sanctions,[4] and narcotics officers generally ignore violations by individual users. The situation is such that if a respected resident of the White House went on television and, stubbing out his cigarette and lighting up a joint, said:

"Well if this is right (holding up the Report of the Second Marijuana Commission), and I believe it is, *this* (pointing to the joint) makes a lot more sense than *that* (the stubbed out cigarette)," it is probable that legislation legalizing marijuana would quickly follow.

But no President of the foreseeable future is likely

to do such a thing unless he is certain more votes will be lost by *not* doing it. Such calculations are always chancy, which means he will do the "safe" thing, i.e., rely upon the advice of the "experts"— those members of the medical profession who claim to be knowledgeable about the effects of drugs. If past experience is any guide, they will maintain that "we don't know enough about this yet, not all the evidence is in," and do so even when there is a millennium of experience behind a drug. And the doctors' motivation for resisting moves which would allow people to do what they will with their own bodies and minds is not a simple, altruistic concern with the people's well-being. It is much more complex, and the first thing to understand is that doctors *love* drugs and, like most lovers, they are jealous and protective of their love. Moreover, they are ardent practitioners of the double standard. As such, they see nothing wrong with flirting or even indulging themselves with choice members of the passing throng; but their beloved must remain pure. When a new drug with wondrous powers comes into the doctor's possession, he falls in love with it and dispenses it for as many reasons as he can. (The only thing exceptional about Freud's love affair with cocaine was the extent and accuracy of his knowledge about its effects.) This eager passing of the drug to other hands in no way sullies its purity, for so long as it remains in the doctor's control all is well. But one of the results of all this love is the rash of drug fads which periodically grip the medical world. Opium, morphine, heroin, cocaine, amphetamines, and tranquilizers were all overprescribed during their careers.[5] And this enthusiasm is infectious. More and more people are exposed to a particular drug and more and more people become knowledgeable about its effects. They learn, for example, that cocaine not only banishes their fatigue and makes them energetic—it also makes them feel *good*. Then they discover that even when they are feeling good a couple of snorts makes them feel *better*. Pretty soon some of them decide it's silly to bother the doctor when all they have to do is step around to the corner drugstore and get whatever they need. After all they don't feel sick, they simply want to feel better.

What has happened is that a growing number of former "patients" no longer need the excuse of some ailment for taking a drug. It makes them feel good and that is excuse enough. Put another way, they are now using the drug for *pleasure*. And at this juncture, the medical community begins to react. People, many people, are taking pleasure with *their* love. Something must be done—ignorant laymen can't be expected to respect the loved one, they will *abuse* it. Dire pronouncements appear concerning the evil effects of the drug: "Nothing so quickly deteriorates its victims or provides so short a route to the insane asylum."[6] Terrible examples are cited: "They give up all that they possess, even indispensable articles of clothing, in order to indulge their mad craving."[7] This makes interesting reading, and the newspapers, always on the lookout for signs of moral decay in the society, gladly print the stuff, and solicit more of the same from like-minded physicians. The clergy and the police, groups who at any given time can be relied upon to announce the approaching moral disintegration of society, happily join the chorus: "Police find criminals favor cocaine to stimulate their 'courage',"[8] and "When cocaine commenced to reach out to his 'boys,' as the Father calls the young men of his parish, he arose to combat it."[9] (As did Samson, to slay the Philistines with the jawbone of an ass.) Politicians react to this pressure and laws are passed restricting the drug. And so it goes.

Of course it doesn't go in quite so straight a line. Some physicians denounce a new drug the moment it is introduced, and some defend it long after the majority of their colleagues have damned it to hell. But once a drug which doesn't enjoy the advantage of being long-established in the culture becomes identified with pleasure, the game is really out of the physician's hands. Its legal life is bound to be short and the execution is a matter of law, the province of politicians who have their own game to play—reelection.

At this stage, therefore, the most important factor in the equation is *who* is using the drug. For traditionally the surest way for a politician to gain votes with an antidrug stand is to tie drug use to some feared and despised group. Since pleasure is sought by all classes, this is never hard to do. The Chinese smoked opium, the blacks snorted cocaine, the Mexican-Americans used marijuana, and the hippies took LSD. In all these cases the politicians, with the aid of the press, identified the drug with the users, and its prohibition was made easy.

But why, for example, should cocaine have been outlawed and not alcohol? After all, far more blacks drank booze than snorted coke. The answer is simply that alcohol has been drunk for so long and by so broad a spectrum of people in this country that its use is considered an established right. (It once *was* prohibited, but the noble experiment was a dismal failure and the law had to be repealed.) Whether it is chewing coca in Peru or drinking alcohol in America, what people have done for a long time they consider their right to keep on doing—and political power never succeeds in abolishing such rights for very long.

With a new drug, the situation is quite different. There is always some resistance to it but if its effects in normal doses are relatively mild, its chances of survival are much better than when its effects in normal doses are relatively strong. When coffee was first introduced to the Arabian peninsula and then later into England, it was the object of fierce denunciations.[10] But it soon received a favorable reception in high places, it seemed innocuous, and it became firmly ensconced in the cultures. Similarly, the more obvious the pleasure a new drug provides, the more likely it is to be repressed. Governments the world over have never been happy about pleasures which take the citizens' minds off work; they are even less happy about pleasures which may affect the users' feelings about those in power. It is, for example, neither whimsy nor a failure to appreciate the effects of such drugs which led governments to suppress marijuana and LSD.

Consciously or unconsciously, they have rightly understood that these drugs are sensitizing agents, the use of which is not in their own self-interest. A person mildly stoned on grass and watching Nixon on TV is much more likely to be appalled by his transparent knavery than one smashed on alcohol, a central nervous system depressant. And someone really stoned on acid would probably have to flee the room, horror-stricken that such a man was our duly elected chief honcho.

Well, enough of theorizing. Take if you will or reject it, but in either case try to hold off your decision until you have read what follows, the details which I believe lend credence to the generalities. For the transformation of cocaine from a "good" drug into an especially dangerous drug does follow, historically, this outline. As usual, however, when you descend from theory to fact, the situation is a bit more complicated.

Following Koller's demonstration of its usefulness as a local anesthetic, cocaine gained acceptance so quickly in the medical world and its nonmedical use spread so rapidly that it seemed as if it would enjoy as long an uncritical run in the West as coca had in the Andes. But cocaine, unlike coca, had never been without its critics. A year after Freud had published his song of praise, Germany's leading morphine addiction specialist published a paper attacking Freud and the notion that cocaine was a cure for morphine addiction.[11] (Freud, by the way, was more pleased than upset by Erlenmeyer's attack. In a letter to a friend he noted that Erlenmeyer's paper "has the advantage of mentioning that it was I who recommended the use of cocaine in cases of morphium addiction, which the people who have confirmed its value there never do."[12]) Then in January of 1886, Obersteiner, who at a medical congress held during the preceding summer had warmly defended Freud and, contra Erlenmeyer, upheld the value of cocaine for withdrawing addicts from morphine, admitted in a paper on intoxication psychoses that "the continued use of cocaine

74

could lead to a delirium tremens very similar to that produced by alcohol."[13] Not long after this, incidents of cocaine "intoxication" were reported from many parts of the world.[14] Then in May of 1886 Erlenmeyer again attacked Freud, this time accusing him of releasing the "third scourge of mankind."[15] A new edition of Erlenmeyer's major work, *On Morphia Addiction,* incorporating his attacks on cocaine and Freud, came out in 1887, at a time when cocaine "addiction" was causing alarm in Germany and everywhere else cocaine was being widely used. By 1891 some 200 cases of cocaine intoxication and 13 deaths from cocaine poisoning had been reported.[16] (How reliable these reports were is difficult to say; but it is interesting that the medical literature of the past few decades contains no reports of deaths among social users.)[17]

That the first strong criticism of cocaine came from the addiction specialists was no accident. Even more than most of their colleagues, the physicians most closely involved in the treatment of opium and morphine addicts were leery of pleasure-producing drugs, no matter how useful they might be. After all, God's Own Medicine, morphine, had been hailed as the savior of mankind, the most useful drug in the doctor's medicine chest. Not only was it the most efficient pain-killer yet devised but it "cured" opium addiction. Give an opium addict morphine and almost always he lost interest in opium. Eventually it was realized that though such treatment usually eliminated an opium addict, it always created a morphine addict. Believing they saw the same pattern developing with cocaine, the addiction specialists were understandably apprehensive.

But their apprehension, expressed in the belief that cocaine was an addictive drug like morphine, only worse, was misplaced, to say the least. True, cocaine was a pleasurable drug—but its pleasures were decidedly different from those of morphine. The one was a central nervous system stimulant, the other a depressant. And unlike the morphinist, the user of cocaine had no need to take increasingly larger doses

75

to get the same effect, and suffered no agonizing withdrawal symptoms when he discontinued cocaine. In short, he was not an addict.[18] So if Erlenmeyer was correct in refuting the claim that cocaine cured opiate addiction, he was guilty of a ludicrous overstatement when he accused Freud of having released the third scourge of humanity. Classifying cocaine a scourge the equal of opium and alcohol was as basic an error of conception as Nixon equating saving his own skin with saving the Presidency. Cocaine neither led to opiate-type addiction nor did habitual use result in the kind of physiological damage associated with alcoholism.[19]

(Strange as it may seem, those who believed cocaine *did* cure opiate addicts were probably less confused about cocaine's action than were their critics. The mechanism of addiction was even less understood then than it is now, and everyone agreed that withdrawal was the key to cure. If an addict could be successfully withdrawn from his drug, then a cure was assured if he had sufficient willpower to stay away from the drug. And since cocaine did in fact help many through the withdrawal period, its advocates were justified in believing it a cure for addiction. Of course they were wrong, but they were wrong because they misunderstood the mechanism of addiction, not because they were advocating one addiction to cure another as their critics charged.)

The failure of cocaine to cure opiate addiction and the fact that some patients found they enjoyed cocaine more than morphine, enlisted some doctors in the anticocaine ranks but the wholesale dispensing of the drug by way of the patent and proprietary medicines enlisted a great many more. For whatever their ideas on cocaine, they took a very dim view of self-medication, a practice which had made America the world's greatest consumer of opium, morphine, and cocaine. Between 1860 and 1911 the population increased by 133 per cent, the consumption of opium by 351 per cent.[20] Turn-of-the-century estimates of opiate addiction ranged from 400,000 to 4,000,000 in a population of 80,000,000.[21] Much of this could be attributed to the vast array of opiate-containing patent medicines consumed by Americans without the benefit of a doctor's advice, but it had been the medical profession's enthusiasm for the opiates which had made them so acceptable to the country and, in turn, so profitable an item for the patent medicine industry.[22] It is not, then, hard to understand why doctors grew apprehensive when cocaine became the rage following their touting it as the new wonder drug and its subsequent exploitation by the patent medicine makers. Their naive enthusiasm for the opiates had led to a great deal of addiction, and the responsibility had been laid at their doorstep in strong terms: "Physicians . . . continually prescribe opium for insufficient causes or without any real excuse."[23]

Was the same thing going to happen with cocaine? If its promotion by the patent medicine people was any indication, it certainly would. The pattern was identical. Few doctors were willing to criticize their colleagues for prescribing too much cocaine, but all doctors could join together in abusing their common enemy, the patent medicine industry, which sold potent drugs to anyone with the money to pay. The pharmacists of the country felt the same way and both groups longed to wean Americans from their reliance on patent medicines. But desire was one thing, practice quite another. The American public seemed willing enough to believe their doctors when the prescribed product made them feel good but, over all, they had little faith in them. They had, indeed, little reason to have faith. The typical doctor practicing in the last third of the nineteenth century was a badly educated incompetent who followed one medical fad after another and knew so little about drugs that he was unable to dispute intelligently the preposterous claims of the patent medicine men.[24] Many had no training to speak of, countless others received their credentials from diploma mills, and even at Harvard the situation was so bad that in 1870 the dean of the Medical School excused the absence of written examinations by explaining that "a majority of the students cannot write well enough."[25]

But if they were not proficient in the written word, they apparently were capable of doing the simple arithmetic which showed that patent medicines claimed many customers who otherwise would be doctors' patients. The pharmacists were equally aware that self-interest demanded something be done and, while the doctors genteelly confined their criticism to pointing out the dangers of addiction and the inherent evils of self-medication, the pharmacists got down to the heart of the matter.

"Do we not recognize that this industry is one of our great enemies, and that there are millions of dollars worth sold all over the country, thus diverting money which rightly belongs to the retail drug trade, in the way of prescriptions and regular drugs?"[26] ("Regular drugs," by the way, included such items as 100 per cent pure cocaine which required no prescription.) A lot of doctors must have cheered when they read this statement made from the podium at the 1893 meeting of the American Pharmaceutical Association, but nothing much came of it. The self-interest which dictated it also militated against any decisive action. For though the speaker quoted understood that he and his fellows would in the long run profit from drastically limiting the number of patent medicines they stocked for sale, the majority of his colleagues couldn't see beyond their immediate self-interest. Patent medicines accounted for a substantial part of their profits and a bird in hand is worth two in the bush.[27] And the most potent voices of the doctors, their medical journals, were similarly chained to short-term interests. The advertisements of the patent medicine industry were their largest source of income and only a handful of the 250 medical journals published in 1900 resisted the medicine manufacturers' demands that plugs for their products "appear disguised as articles or editorials."[28] Indeed more than a few of these journals were owned by the manufacturers themselves.[29] Even the *Journal of the American Medical Association,* the most prestigious of the publications, was filled with dubious patent medicine ads and the claims of medical quacks as late as 1905.[30] And though on more than one occasion the AMA's leaders responded to criticism of this practice by trying to eliminate such material from the *Journal,* each attempted reform was abandoned in the face of growing publishing deficits.[31] Money talks, and the patent medicine industry had the money.

Meanwhile, however, a new body of critics, the agricultural chemists, began to make themselves heard. Initially, they had confined their investigations to the production and marketing of foods but, following the example of their acknowledged spokesman, Dr. Harvey Wiley, chief chemist of the Department of Agriculture, they broadened their inquiries to include patent medicines. In 1903, Wiley set up within the Bureau of Chemistry, a laboratory devoted to the analysis of proprietary remedies and, more importantly, continued to stump the country telling Americans they were being defrauded both in the foods they ate and the medicines they took.[32] He was an eloquent, forceful speaker and, given his position, his criticisms carried the weight of official government pronouncements. The press treated him as an oracle and when *Collier's* magazine hired Samuel Hopkins Adams to write an exposé of the patent medicine industry in 1905, Adams immediately went to Wiley, who gave him a good grounding in the field and provided him with leads.[33] Adams had a genius for investigative reporting, and his articles, packed with revelatory detail and appearing as they did in a magazine of *Collier's* prestige and circulation, made a devastating impact on the public, the AMA— (which between 1905 and 1912 issued 500,000 low-priced copies of *The Great American Fraud*),[34] and the Congress which under the pressure of the Adams pieces, Upton Sinclair's exposé of the meat-packing business, the lobbying of the AMA, and the prodding of Dr. Wiley, finally got round to passing the Pure Food and Drug Act of 1906, and with it put an end to the indiscriminate use of opiates, cocaine, and other drugs in patent medicines.

79

All this was of decided benefit to the country's well-being, but with respect to the question at hand—how cocaine came to be considered an especially dangerous drug—it was only a preliminary, if necessary step. The war against patent medicines was also, of course, a war against those particular ones which contained cocaine, but it was a war fought by its physician and pharmacist combatants essentially for self-interest; and it is hard to see how self-interest led to such statements as "there is nothing that we can do for the confirmed user of the drug, the best thing for the cocaine fiend is to let him die,"[35] and "the dull white crystals . . . contain the most insidious effects of any known drug."[36] Hard to see, that is, unless these favorites of the newspapers had abandoned all pretense to being men of science concerned with matters of fact, and were now bent on establishing themselves as the courted mouthpieces of interests best known for their antipathy to fact. For with the exception of the articles written by those addiction specialists who, in their eagerness to denounce anyone who advocated cocaine as a cure for opiate addiction, were capable of saying and believing that cocaine was even worse than morphine, there is nothing in the medical literature of the time to support the view that cocaine was the most insidious of known drugs. Very few doctors reported any difficulty in withdrawing a patient from cocaine. On the contrary, almost all reported it was easy. As Lucius P. Brown, the Food and Drugs Commissioner of Tennessee, flatly stated in an article on the enforcement of the state's antinarcotics law:

'I want to call particular attention here to the fact that the habitual use of cocaine is not a disease, but a habit, inasmuch as it does not produce such toxemias as are consequent on the use of morphine; therefore its abrupt withdrawal results in no such untoward consequences as with the latter drug. No provision [for allowing addicts to get their drugs on prescription], therefore, need be made for the relief of persons [habituated] to it."[37]

80

(Brown had earlier made a point of reminding physicians that opiate addiction was a disease, that abrupt withdrawal caused unnecessary suffering without curing the disease, and that addicts should be treated as patients and not criminals. Hence, the issuing of prescriptions which allowed them to legally procure the drugs they needed.)

Whatever else it may have been, cocaine was assuredly not the most insidious of known drugs. And since the *facts* about its effects could hardly have created such a fantasy, something else must have been responsible. It shouldn't surprise anyone to learn that once cocaine became firmly associated in the nation's consciousness with blacks, the black-menace fantasies jumping through the American psyche found a further outlet in fantasies about the menace of cocaine. Or, blacks used cocaine, blacks were a menace, therefore cocaine was a menace. A syllogism which would assure you a failing grade in logic, but fantasy is not constrained by reason.

The minor premise, however, was correct. Blacks *did* use cocaine. Like everyone else in the country they used patent medicines and some found they preferred the ones based on cocaine to those built on the opiates. Moreover, plantation overseers and gang bosses, like the Spaniards with the Incas, had discovered that things went better with coke. They kept a supply on hand and passed it out to the workers.[38] As a means of keeping the hands happy and insuring more productivity, it was both efficient and cheap. A shrewd boss doling out one-quarter gram a day per man could keep sixteen workers happy and more productive for a full seven days on a single ounce. With cocaine selling at $2.50 the ounce, he could hardly go wrong. And Southern blacks also bought cocaine on their own. Some historians believe the blacks of the South turned to cocaine when most of the states passed legislation which effectively barred them from access to alcohol.[39] Some undoubtedly did get into cocaine in this way, but the majority began buying cocaine for the same reason as their white counterparts—they liked it.

However cocaine use started among Southern blacks, articles began to appear on the subject expressing more than a little concern. In 1898, the *Medical News* carried a story which especially associated cocaine abuse with Southern blacks.[40] In 1900 an editorial in the *Journal of the American Medical Association* told its readers: "The Negroes in some parts of the South are reported as being addicted to a new form of vice— that of cocaine 'snuffing' or the 'coke habit'!"[41] By 1902 enough attention had been given the subject that the *British Medical Journal* printed a piece entitled, "The Cocaine Habit Among Negroes," in which it was revealed that "On many Yazoo plantations this year the negroes refused to work unless they could be assured that there was some place in the neighborhood where they could get cocaine, and it is said that some planters kept the drug in stock among the plantation supplies, and issued regular rations of cocaine just as they used to issue regular rations of whiskey."[42]

This use of cocaine by Southern blacks coincided with that period when the white South was in the last stages of dismantling the remnants of Reconstruction. Legal segregation, voting laws shaped to deprive blacks of any share in the political process, and lynchings to impress them of the realities of life in the South, were all at their peak during the last decade of the nineteenth century. Quite naturally, the whites responsible for these actions were a bit uneasy, and their uneasiness was not lessened by the generally held belief that cocaine would act as a "spur to violence against whites."[43] It was bad enough thinking about how ordinary blacks might rebel and strike back at their oppressors; but the idea that blacks filled with cocaine might be doing the striking was apparently insupportable. Anecdotal material from the region "often told of superhuman strength, cunning, and efficiency resulting from cocaine."[44]

Newspaper articles appeared linking cocaine with black violence. In 1903, the *New York Tribune* printed a statement by one Colonel Watson of Georgia alerting the country to the dangers of allowing blacks to use cocaine. According to him, Atlanta was a hotbed of black "coke" use and he urged that legal action be taken to stop the sale of Coca-Cola. (The company responded by voluntarily eliminating cocaine from the drink that same year.) The colonel was convinced that "many of the horrible crimes committed in the Southern States by the colored people can be traced directly to the cocaine habit."[45] This ploy, the association of cocaine with crimes allegedly committed by blacks, became immensely popular.

For example, the police chief of the District of Columbia, concerned about black crime, testified that cocaine was the greatest drug menace of all.[46] And the police chief of Atlanta, even more concerned, maintained that 70 per cent of the crimes committed in his city could be traced to cocaine.[47] The equating of blacks and cocaine with crime was so firmly established by 1910 that when Dr. Christopher Koch, the leader of a Philadelphia crusade against the drug, in testimony before a congressional committee holding hearings on the possibility of drafting a federal anti-narcotics law, pointed out the dangers the country faced at the hands of cocaine-crazed Southern blacks, his testimony went unchallenged.[48] Dr. Koch was later quoted as asserting that "Most of the attacks upon white women of the South are the direct result of a cocaine-crazed Negro brain,"[49] a piece of nonsense which, so far as I can determine, also went unchallenged. But by this time the chance of common sense's intervening and asserting facts about the effects of cocaine couldn't be said to exist. Once the equation, blacks plus cocaine equals raped white women, had taken hold in the national consciousness and the deepest sexual fears of white America stirred, any argument likely to aid in the total outlawing of cocaine was both believed and welcomed.

Of course all these fearmongering fantasies were just that, fantasies, and nothing more. Neither the police chiefs, the doctors, nor anyone else who made these statements offered any *evidence* to back them up. That such evidence didn't exist was hardly a problem. Cocaine was a convenient explanation of "crime waves,"[50] a way of explaining white fears of blacks without having to face why they were really feared, and that seemed to be enough for the country. It was all very like the heyday of the late Senator Joe McCarthy, a gifted liar given to waving sheets of paper in the air which allegedly contained the names of large numbers of Communists being harbored by the traitorous State Department. He never showed anyone the names (he didn't have any), the number count changed from day to day, but no matter, most of the country believed him. He became, on the strength of this simple tactic, a power great enough to frighten into silence almost all who opposed him. And McCarthy was playing on only the ideological fears of Americans —God knows what he might have accomplished had he been able to equate reds with blacks, and mined the deep wells of sexual and racial fear.

What McCarthy failed to do and what the denouncers of blacks and cocaine succeeded in doing resulted in some truly marvelous hyperbole on how cocaine affected blacks—some of which, had it been taken seriously, would have assured a run on cocaine by every gangster, police department, and army in the world. The best effort I have encountered, a milestone in exaggeration, appeared in *The New York Times* of February 8, 1914. Entitled "Negro Cocaine 'Fiends' Are A New Southern Menace," and written by Edward Huntington Williams, M.D., it summarizes most of the myths associated with black crime and cocaine. And though it conspicuously omits any direct reference to "cocaine-crazed blacks" raping white women, the omission is probably more due to the fact that he was writing for the august *Times* than to any lack of belief on Dr. Williams's part. Or perhaps he didn't see any need to repeat such well-known, generally accepted material—blacks raped white women whenever they got the chance, everyone knew that. But if Dr. Williams refused to cater to the prurient interests, he certainly didn't shy from the spectacular. Here is a sampling of his wares, from the simple wild exaggeration to the unbelievable:[51]

—"There is no escaping the conviction that drug taking has become a race menace in certain regions south of the line."

—"He [the cocaine fiend] imagines that he hears people taunting or abusing him, and this often incites homicidal attacks upon innocent and unsuspecting victims."

—"Stories of cocaine orgies, followed by wholesale murders, seem like lurid journalism of the yellowest variety. But in point of fact there was nothing 'yellow' about . . . these reports. Nine men killed in Mississippi on one occasion by crazed cocaine takers, five in North Carolina, three in Tennessee—these are facts that need no imaginative coloring."

(Or wouldn't if they *were* facts. But I have found nothing in the historical record to indicate that they are other than Dr. Williams's unsupported assertion; which, given his gullibility, is hardly enough.)

—"The list of dangerous effects produced by cocaine . . . is certainly long enough. But there is another, and a most important one. This is a temporary steadying of the nervous and muscular system, so as to increase, rather than interfere with good marksmanship. . . . The record of the 'cocaine nigger' near Asheville, who dropped five men dead in their tracks, using only one cartridge for each, offers evidence that is sufficiently convincing."

And, as if things weren't bad enough with black cocaine fiends picking off innocent bystanders with superhuman accuracy, there was the added problem of the police not having sufficient firepower to stop them:

—"The drug produces several other conditions that make the 'fiend' a peculiarly dangerous criminal. One of these conditions is a temporary immunity to shock—a resistance to the 'knock down' effects of fatal wounds. Bullets fired into vital parts, that would drop a sane man in his tracks, fail to check the 'fiend'—fail to stop his rush or weaken his attack.

"A recent experience of Chief of Police Lyerly of Asheville N.C., illustrates this particular phase of cocainism. The Chief was informed that a hitherto inoffensive negro was 'running amuck' in a cocaine frenzy. . . . Knowing that he must kill the man or be killed himself, the Chief drew his revolver [a heavy army model . . . large enough to kill any game in America], placed the muzzle over the negro's heart and fired—'intending to kill him right quick'—but the shot did not even stagger the man. And a second shot that pierced the arm and entered the chest had just as little effect in stopping the negro or checking his attack."

Chief Lyerly, however, won the day when he remembered the teachings of his boyhood—that a nigger's head is not a vital part—and "finished the man with his club." And he learned a lesson: the next day he got himself a revolver of heavier caliber. Police officers all over the South did likewise.[52]

(Policemen looking for an excuse to acquire heavier weapons have become an American tradition. In the 1960's they got themselves armored vehicles, automatic rifles, and the like ostensibly in response to the likelihood of armed insurrection in the black ghettos. A bit later they upped their firepower again, this time ostensibly in response to the "menace" posed by the "radical" elements of the antiwar movement. Nothing happened then or later to justify such weaponry, but the police still have it, and under Nixon's Law Enforcement Assistance Agency policies are getting still more. The latest, and silliest, escalation I'm aware of is the arming of the New York State Police with .357 magnums, "capable of blowing apart the engine block of a car," because the troopers "didn't feel safe with their old .38s." According to the radio news broadcast which carried this information, the troopers had killed quite a few things over the past year but only three of them were human, most of the rest being stray or injured deer.[53] (I suppose the deer were too dangerous to face with a measly .38. Maybe they were all coked up.)

Not only did white fears provide the black cocaine users with imaginary attributes, but there was also a widely held belief that cocaine was especially suited to blacks and that its use was more prevalent among them than other groups. The direct evidence to support such beliefs does not exist. Indeed at least one report from the South indicated that cocaine use among blacks was considerably less than among whites.[54] However, the replies to questionnaires sent out by the American Pharmaceutical Association's Committee on the Acquirement of the Drug Habit to physicians and pharmacists in 1902 and 1903 do indicate a marked increase in cocaine sales over previous years, especially to blacks. Nothing in the Report of the Committee indicates, of course, anything to the effect that cocaine was especially suitable for blacks, nor is there any indication that cocaine was more prevalent among blacks than other groups. The Committee in fact took care to note that cocaine use cut across all sectors of society.[55] The fact is that all such attempts to estimate drug use, then or now, are, at best, very rough, educated guesses and usually a good deal less than educated.

(In a speculative vein, it strikes me that the stimulant quality of cocaine may well have made it more appealing than the opiates to those who had to work hard

87

to feed themselves—the blacks and the lower-class whites. Cocaine would help them work harder, the opiates would not.)

But the belief that cocaine was especially suited to blacks (and lower-class whites) was not founded either on facts or speculations based on the effects of the drug. So far as I can tell, it received its credibility from the popular notion that the poor were stupid and/or lazy:

"The negro drug 'fiend' uses cocaine almost exclusively. This preference is not explained by the difference in the effects of the two drugs, morphine and cocaine, but rather in the manner that each drug may be taken. Morphine . . . taken hypodermically . . . requires special apparatus, a liquid solution of the drug, and a somewhat complicated process of preparation. Cocaine, on the other hand, can be taken in the dry form by the simple process of sniffing into the nose like an ordinary pinch of snuff."[56]

And from another author,

"In its use, requiring as it does none of the sometimes elaborate paraphernalia associated with the abuse of opium and morphine, it appeals to the most wretched classes of drug victims in the cities, to the negro field hands of the South, as well as to the tramp in his 'jungle'."[57]

Of course, these and other quotations to the same effect can be interpreted in quite another fashion, namely, that the poor couldn't afford a syringe and thus had to make do with cocaine. But apart from certain terms (elaborate, complicated, simple) and an over-all tone which imply that it was the process rather than the cost of using the opiates which stopped the poor, this interpretation simply doesn't stand up for a number of reasons. In the first place, people take drugs for their effects and they are not going to use a central nervous system stimulant if they want its opposite. Moreover, though the typical opiate addict of 1900 was middle-class or affluent, there were plenty of poor ones, and if some of them could afford the apparatus why not the others? And one could simply eat or drink the stuff, a syringe wasn't essential.

In any event, whether they used it because they were poor, stupid, lazy, or preferred it to other drugs, the ordinary cocaine user was also unrefined: "A . . . catarrh snuff tube and bulb is all the apparatus required even by the nicer victims. The mass simply snuff the stuff up from the palm or from between thumb and finger."[58]

In addition to the blacks and poor whites, another less than highly esteemed group became identified with cocaine use—criminals. Among policemen, the special fondness criminals had for cocaine was an article of faith as unquestioned as purity of the Holy Mother. Criminals as a matter of course took cocaine to stimulate their "courage."[59] "Lying and stealing are the least of the crimes he is ready to commit when under the influence, and, in the majority of cases, his nature becomes brutalized and changed for the worse."[60] And "police experience with criminals revealed that cocaine was the drug usually taken by gunmen."[61]

All the elements needed to insure cocaine's outlaw status were present by the first years of the twentieth century: it had become widely used as a pleasure drug, and doctors warned of the dangers attendant on indiscriminate sale and use; it had become identified with despised or poorly regarded groups—blacks, lower-class whites, and criminals; it had not been long enough established in the culture to insure its survival; and it had not, though used by them, become identified with the elite, thus losing what little chance it had of weathering the storm of criticism. Such statements as "there is little doubt that every Jew peddler in the South carries the stuff," printed in the prestigious *New York Times* were hardly calculated to lessen the demands that cocaine be banned.[62]

With so much going against it, it is not surprising that cocaine was virtually outlawed in America several years before morphine and heroin, drugs which, though used by all classes of society, were more identified with the affluent than the poor. But one opiate, opium, was identified with a despised group; and, since just as the medical profession rarely acknowledges the harmful effects of certain drugs until a significant level of pleasure use has been attained, the government rarely enacts restrictive legislation until a drug is identified with racial minorities or the poor, it might be instructive, before going into the details of the anti-cocaine laws to review briefly how opium was banned long before its more powerful offspring, morphine and heroin.

Opium was the traditional drug of China. When the Chinese were brought to America as cheap labor to help build the railroads during the great westward expansion of the mid 1800s, they carried their opium habit with them. In due time they formed a surplus labor pool and, much worse, an exceedingly cheap surplus labor pool which threatened the security of the American worker.[63] The racial prejudice then directed against them was a natural outcome, but little was ever said about the real reason they were so disliked—the economic competition they represented. Instead, time and time again, their opium-smoking was cited as a threat to the American way of life. Wild stories appeared in the press about opium being used to entice young white maidens to a fate worse than death, etc., etc.[64] Inevitably, opium was banned. Smoking opium used by the Chinese, that is. The opium-filled patent medicines much loved by white America were not affected. The Chinese being mainly established in the West, the Western states led the way. Nevada passed a law prohibiting the sale of opiates for nonmedical purposes in 1877, and by 1891 most of the Western states had enacted statutes prohibiting opium smoking.[65]

Legislation against cocaine was equally prompt and even more widespread. In 1887, Oregon prohibited the sale of cocaine without a doctor's prescription.[66] Montana did likewise in 1889, New York in 1893, Colorado and Illinois in 1897, Arizona and Arkansas in 1899, and Mississippi in 1900.[67] (Again, none of these laws affected patent medicines containing cocaine. Unlike the targets of this legislation, the patent medicine industry was rich and powerful.) By 1914, and prior to the enactment of the federal Harrison Narcotics Act, forty-six states had passed some form of legislation designed to regulate the use and distribution of cocaine.[68] That cocaine was considered *the* dangerous drug is evident from the fact that by 1914 only twenty-nine states had passed similar legislation against the opiates.[69]

The Harrison Narcotics Act of 1914—the basis, until 1970, of all federal laws controlling dangerous drugs—was the first federal antidrug law in the nation's history and, like the state laws preceding it, its provisions incorporated the prevailing belief that cocaine was the most dangerous of the pleasure drugs. Under Harrison, possession of cocaine by an unregistered person—that is, by anyone not licensed to distribute or use it for medical purposes—though not in itself a crime, was considered presumptive evidence of a violation of the Act. Those convicted of illegally distributing or using cocaine were punishable by fines of up to $2000, a prison term of up to five years, or both. Consistent with the policy established by the states, medicinal preparations containing small amounts of opium or its derivatives (usually morphine and heroin)—the drugs most used by the population as a whole—were exempt from the provisions of the Act. But no preparation containing any amount of cocaine —the presumed favorite of the blacks, the poor, and the criminals—and sold by "Jew peddlers"—was exempt.[70]

In 1919, the Harrison Act was amended to provide for tighter controls on cocaine and opium.[71] The government was once again trying to come down hard on minorities.

Then in 1922, the Congress amended the Narcotic

91

Drugs Import and Export Act which had been passed, along with Harrison, in 1914, to ban the importation of cocaine and coca leaves. Coca leaves could be brought in but only in those amounts needed to manufacture cocaine for medical purposes. For the first time, cocaine was clearly, and mistakenly, classed as a narcotic drug. Penalties for violating the law were more stringent than any in prior federal statutes. Instead of a fine, or imprisonment, or both, violators were fined up to $5000 *and* imprisoned for up to ten years.[72]

Congress, in its attempt to regulate and prohibit the distribution, sale, and use of drugs, kept on passing new laws and amending old ones—usually for the sole purpose of making the penalties harsher—until 1970 when it enacted the Comprehensive Drug Abuse Prevention and Control Act of 1970, which repealed all existing federal drug laws. Cocaine is still misclassified as a narcotic drug, and is listed under Schedule II with those drugs having a currently accepted medical use but a "high potential for abuse that can lead to severe psychological or physical dependence." As one would expect, the new Act carries stiffer penalties than the old ones. Prior to 1970, for example, though unauthorized possession of cocaine was presumptive evidence of a violation, it was not in itself a crime; under the new Act, mere possession is a felony. Also anyone who illegally manufactures, dispenses, distributes, or possesses cocaine with intent to sell is punishable by a prison term of not more than 15 years, a fine of up to $25,000, or both. If the violator has a prior drug conviction or sells to someone under twenty-one years of age, the maximum penalties are doubled. Any violator who is considered an established drug dealer and classified as a "dangerous special drug offender" receives a minimum sentence of ten years and a fine up to $100,000 for the first conviction. A subsequent conviction doubles the penalties. Possession of cocaine for personal use is punishable by a maximum of one year in prison, a fine of up to $5000, or both.[73]

Some states provide even harsher penalties. What

can get you 15 years if busted by a federal narc, can bring you a mandatory life sentence without parole if busted by a New York narc. (See Appendix II for a rundown on the current legal situation.)

Like most other pleasure drugs, cocaine became a banned substance not because objective tests showed it to be dangerous, but because of grossly mistaken beliefs about its effects which grew primarily from its association in the public mind with feared or despised minority groups. That it further came to be regarded as an especially dangerous drug, *the* most dangerous drug, is reflected by the manner in which it was treated under a variety of antidrug statutes. To briefly sum up this latter point: (1) by 1914, forty-six states had passed legislation restricting the sale and use of cocaine, but only twenty-nine had done so respecting the opiates; (2) more stringent penalties were frequently provided for cocaine offenders than for other drug violators. For example, illegal sale of opium or heroin was punishable in 1914 in New York as a misdemeanor under the public health law, whereas illegal sale of cocaine was punishable as a felony under the penal law;[74] and (3) cocaine was singled out for special treatment in federal laws. Under Harrison, for example, preparations containing small amounts of opiates were exempt, but no preparation containing any amount of cocaine was exempt.

If any further proof is needed of cocaine's unique status, consider the fact that it has been willfully misclassified in federal and most state laws as a narcotic drug since at least 1922. I say willfully misclassified, since the government drug experts knew very well it was a stimulant drug and not the opposite, a narcotic drug. Classifying it as a narcotic, however, afforded distinct propaganda advantages. (PROPAGANDA: (1) the art of lying, by either commission or omission, for the purpose of influencing opinion; (2) a technique used by governments, corporations, and assorted scoundrels to keep citizens from learning the truth.)[75] The vast majority of drug horror tales carried in the newspapers and magazines referred only to "narcotics" and seldom mentioned specific drugs. By calling cocaine a narcotic the government anticocaine propagandists reaped the advantage of having all the drug-innocent citizens associate these frightening stories of narcotic addiction with cocaine as well as with the opiates which the stories, in fact, usually were about. Moreover, during the first decades of this century, a sizable proportion of the public undoubtedly believed that the opiates induced violence (see, e.g., Sax Rohmer's Fu Manchu novels) and cocaine sedation (Conan Doyle in *A Scandal in Bohemia*). And by misclassifying cocaine as a narcotic, the antidrug people could take advantage of this misapprehension.

This mistaken association of cocaine with the opiates had a lighter side. It could be credited, if you appreciate unintentional comedy, with some real treats. The funniest example I have come across is a 1917 production of the Provincetown Players entitled *Cocaine* (A Play in One Act), by Pendleton King, which would have been more properly called *Morphine* or *Heroin* insofar as its two characters exhibit the addiction and craving common to opiate users and not to cocaine users. Anyway, the play is set in the run-down Bowery room shared by Joe, an ex-prizefighter, and Nora, a former "lady" whose love of dope has brought her low. It is 4 A.M. and Joe is alone, waiting for Nora who is uptown picking pockets to raise enough money to buy what they need. Nora enters the room looking dejected. She hasn't managed to lift a thing. Joe groans that they've been four whole days "widout de stuff."

Nora: I wouldn't have believed I could go so long.
Joe: We're up against it.
Nora: I know we are.
Joe: I wish we could get a good old sniff, and forget our troubles tonight.

Joe then suggests that if he agrees to the landlady's

94

sexual demands, the lusty woman will give them cocaine. She's got lots of it. Nora gets hysterical . . .

> Joe: If I was able to do any kind of work it'd
> be different. But de stuff's got me. . . . I
> don't see why you kick on one old measly
> landlady. . . . I ain't going to leave you.
> But I gotta have de stuff, that's all. I've gone
> without it four days now.

Nora understands needing to have "de stuff"; she feels
the same way; but rather than see Joe prostitute himself she'll commit suicide. Joe objects for a while (the
play must last the one act), and then his nobler
instincts prevail and he agrees to join her. They'll both
commit suicide. They close the window, turn on the
gas, and lie down on the bed to meet death together.
Unfortunately the meter has run out and they don't
have a quarter to start it up again. Curtain.[76]

Levity aside, cocaine is *still* classed as a narcotic
drug under federal and most state laws despite the
fact that (a) it is not, and that (b) one would be hard
pressed to locate a current government publication
on drugs which fails to recognize this fact. This misclassification is not merely a case of one government
hand not knowing what the other is doing; it has
serious practical consequences. To begin with, a narcotics classification allows the courts to impose harsher
sentences than would otherwise be permissible. And
secondly, this deliberate and long-perpetuated error
has led not only the populace at large to identify
cocaine with the truly addictive drugs such as heroin
and the reams of adverse publicity received by these
drugs, but has implanted the same misconception in
the minds of judges—much to the detriment of de-
fendants and the sensible administration of justice.
For example, in a recent cocaine case tried before the
United States District Court in Massachusetts, the judge
explained the basis for the sentence he handed out
in the following terms:

"The reason for the sentence of the Court is simply the word cocaine. That is the one—that is the explanation. Hard narcotics in my opinion demand hard sentences. . . . Anyone who facilitates the transaction in the hard narcotics—and I consider that cocaine is a hard narcotic—has to be made a lesson of, to cut down on the traffic, to cut down on relatively innocent persons like yourselves, who get caught up in the drug subculture. . . . It is not just a question of your welfare as much as it is a question of the welfare of young people in this community who, but for jail sentences of this type will be introduced to these narcotics, may become addicted to these narcotics, and in my view it is essential to take these harsh steps to endeavour to bring the community out of this scourge."[77]

5

The People's Friend Becomes the Rich Man's High

Trying to ascertain with any degree of accuracy just who did what, and how much they did, is the major problem of any illicit drug scholar. Once a drug is driven underground, there cannot be any reliable statistics. As Alfred Lindesmith put it, "When addiction became a criminal act, counting addicts posed much the same difficulties that would be encountered in a census of racketeers."[1]

When the drug in question doesn't produce addiction of the opiate kind, the problem is even greater. For the only data on drug use in general comes from law enforcement departments, the various agencies which treat addicts, the hospitals, private doctors, and individual drug users. The accounts of only this last group are of much value in determining what was happening with cocaine. For cocaine users, unless they are also opiate users, do not come to addiction centers, hospitals, and the like seeking treatment. They do not suffer withdrawal symptoms when deprived of their drug and hence have little if any reason to seek treatment. And since, unlike the opiates, cocaine is not a drug which compels the user to desperate measures to replenish his supply, the police seldom come in contact with a cocaine user unless he is also a dealer.

The newspapers, from which one might expect to gain some idea as to what is going on from day to day in a society, not only usually failed to specify the drug which had been used, sold, or confiscated but, then as now, were much more interested in splashy stories on the arrest of "big" dealers and "huge caches" of "narcotics" than in the doings of ordinary drug users. Occasionally, as in "Seize 'Coke King' and $50,000 Drugs," a *New York Times* headline of 1924,[2] the specific drug was identified; and sometimes the details revealed both the drug involved and the police habit of puffing minor arrests into major ones. For example: "Dr. Simon and a Detective Arrest the 'Cocaine Kid' After a Long Hunt" was the headline, and Dr. Carleton Simon, as any reader of this 1921 edition of the *Times* knew, was Special Deputy Police Commissioner in charge of the Narcotics Squad. The reader might therefore be excused for believing that any dealer personally arrested by the Special Deputy Commissioner after a long hunt was pretty high up in the ranks. But whatever else he was, Dr. Simon was a moralist who couldn't refrain from the telling detail, a habit which usually radically deflated the importance of his arrests. According to him, the Kid (officially known as The Cocaine Kid of Broome Street) had done well in his trade: "The boy has made enough money selling drugs in the last six months to buy several diamond rings and pins, a new automobile of one of the expensive makes, and to become familiar with the amusements of the older men who taught him how to sell drugs." The Kid, who was sixteen and wise to the ways of the police, "offered his captors two diamond rings, a diamond pin and $50 in cash if they would let him escape."[3] But not wise enough. He should have known you can't bribe a Deputy Commissioner in the presence of a working cop, and vice versa. To say nothing of the fact that if they were looking for a bribe they wouldn't have gone after him but his bosses, who surely could have come up with more than $50 cash.

Such stories appeared regularly from 1915 through the early 1930s, and the fact that they usually referred simply to "dope" or "narcotics" reflects how happily the press played along with the fantasies of the police. Both sides were far more interested in creating drama than in reporting fact. And who can blame them? Facts are either scarce or grubby in this area, and fantasies plentiful. The typical drug arrestee is some poor junkie selling on the street to support his habit. This doesn't make very exciting reading nor does it enhance the brave image of the police. Far better then, that every small-time dealer and junkie be raised to a status befitting the needs of the press and the police, needs which have remained pretty constant since the Harrison Act of 1914.

Making all due allowance for a flashier, more care-free era, what the late Wolcott Gibbs wrote about the press of the 1920s is essentially true today: "The intense melodrama of the twenties accustomed people to the idea of an aristocracy of crime, to a super-heated vision of America ruled by an outlaw nobility of vast and incalculable powers. Beer barons and vice lords were a dime a dozen; almost every thug was at least a king. In New York there were kings of vice, poultry, dope, fur, policy, and artichokes, to mention a few, and each of them commanded a band of desperadoes capable of dealing with the United States Marines. It was wonderful."[4]

Indeed it was, and still is. No current reader of the daily press can have failed to encounter dozens of stories on multimillion-dollar drug seizures, the arrests of assorted kingpins of the drug trade, and the busting up of vast drug rings said to be responsible for some large percentage of the drugs circulating in the country. In the early stages of such reading the average reader may have given a sigh of relief and muttered "well, that takes care of that!"; as time goes on, and the stories are repeated month to month and year to year, even the most stolid believer in the wisdom and virtue of our guardians of liberty must begin to wonder: How many "major" drug rings can there be? how many "Mr. Bigs?" Only God knows, for the police seldom apprehend any one above the middle level of dealing, and dealers don't list themselves in the Yellow Pages. When and if the narcs do manage to break up a truly top-level operation—and though there probably aren't as many as they have *already* eradicated, there are more than a few such operations —the press will be hard put to describe it adequately. They and the narcs have previously reported the "No. 1 Heroin Ring . . . Broken"—will they be witty enough to say "*Another* No. 1 Heroin Ring Broken," or sly enough to print "*The* No. 1 Heroin Ring Broken," or will they come down to earth and simply report a "Big Heroin Operation Broken?"

Moreover if one were to take seriously the antidrug literature of any period, it would seem as if hardly anyone used a given nasty substance except those scapegoats who had been identified as its prime users and a menace to every law-abiding decent citizen. But though cocaine came to be considered especially dangerous because it was believed to be the preferred drug of the blacks, the poor, and the criminals, the use of cocaine was hardly confined to these classes. If anything, the middle- and upper-income groups of the country were more into it than anyone else. For cocaine was first extensively used in America in the treatment of opiate addiction, and the typical addict of the period was white and affluent. And when physicians became enthusiastic over cocaine's usefulness as a tonic suitable for all those afflicted with that tired, run-down feeling, the beneficiaries of this new excitement were obviously their patients, few of whom were likely to be really poor.

Enthusiasm for cocaine's stimulant properties was expressed very early in the game. The 1881 statement of Dr. H. F. Stimmel of Chattanooga, Tennessee, was not unusual: "to say that I am surprised and astonished at the wonderful, and almost incredible effects of that new remedy as a nervous stimulant would not adequately express my appreciation of it."[5] Dr. Stimmel was obviously dipping into the cocaine jar himself— as were many of his colleagues. A 1903 report lamented that "many of the leading lights of the medical profession . . . become slaves to a vice [cocaine] which they are supposed to combat."[6] Whether they were slaves or not is debatable, but certainly they and the rest of the medical profession were instrumental in getting cocaine into the hands of the professional and moneyed classes. This same report remarks on how lawyers and preachers took cocaine in order to be "bright"[7]; and goes on to say that one of the reasons for the spread of the drug habit was the belief among physicians that they could build a profitable practice by showing their patients the relaxing or pleasurable effects to be had from one hyperdermic injection.[8] As any modern Dr. Feelgood can testify, this belief was well founded.

As a result then of their ability to consult doctors, either professionally or as friends, the relatively well-to-do were probably the first class of Americans to use cocaine extensively. And it seems at least equally plausible that after cocaine was outlawed and obtainable only on a doctor's prescription or from an illicit dealer, its use became even more the prerogative of those with money. The white poor and the blacks were not in general likely to have been able to afford the new black market prices, and they certainly weren't in the position to pay a doctor for a prescription. Indeed very few of them ever went to a doctor for any reason. This is not to say that once cocaine was prohibited the lower classes were cut off from it completely; it is only to say their ease of access was greatly reduced, while the financially better off were not seriously inconvenienced. As Dr. Ernest Bishop, one of the nation's more intelligent drug authorities, said in 1916, when those who could afford to visit doctors could still get a prescription for cocaine or the opiates, the number of persons of the "upper world" who used habit-forming drugs was "legion," and "they included judges, physicians, lawyers, and ministers."[9]

Though Dr. Bishop did not specify which habit-forming drugs were being used by the legions of the upper world, it is justifiable to assume that cocaine was prominent among them. Most doctors, including Dr. Bishop, believed that cocaine was a habit-forming drug which led to addiction. And both doctors and the press, especially after the Harrison Act of 1914, referred to drugs and addiction in very general, unspecific terms. Addiction figures published at the time included cocaine "addicts" as well as opiate addicts, but they were usually lumped together under a single heading. For example, Dr. Charles Terry, in his capacity as health officer of Jacksonville, Florida, was cited in a Treasury Department Report as having recorded "887 addicts in that city in 1913."[10] When Dr. Terry used this figure in his 1924 classic, *The Opium Problem,* the careful reader could discover that Jacksonville in 1913 had 541 known opiate addicts and, listed in a footnote, 346 cocaine users.[11]

Careful reading, however, is only occasionally of value when one turns to the newspapers in the hope of getting information on the social patterns of cocaine use. In the first place, most of those arrested for drug law violations in earlier times were, as in 1974, on the lowest rungs of the social ladder—street dealers, shady druggists, and their poorer customers. The professional and moneyed classes who were able to get their drugs from the doctors were protected both by the law and their positions. One does not encounter Dr. Bishop's "judges, physicians, lawyers, and ministers" in the pages of the daily papers. (Although between 1914 and 1938 approximately 25,000 physicians were charged under the Harrison Act for illegally prescribing or supplying drugs, and some 3,000 ended up in jail, the names of their clients were rarely mentioned—though one must presume that most of them were regular patients and thus not poor.[12]) But even had every class of drug user been equally liable to arrest, trying to ascertain the specific drug they were using is almost always an exercise in futility. I have read every drug story published in *The New York Times* between 1908 and 1936, and would have read every one prior to 1908 and many after 1936 had I not become discouraged. For in the great preponderance of cases no reference to specific drugs can be found. The terms "drugs," "narcotics," "addicts," "addiction," and occasionally "dope" as in "dope fiends" are sprinkled liberally throughout the stories, but one seldom sees "opium," "morphine," "heroin," or "cocaine."

Contrary to what we have learned over the years about the effects of drug laws, namely, that people don't stop using simply because the law says they should, at least one report claims that the number of upper-class cocaine users dropped off after the enactment of the Harrison Act. "Drug Addiction: Analysis of 147 cases at the Philadelphia General Hospital," a study by two of the hospital's doctors on admissions between 1914 and 1916 of 101 opiate addicts and 47 cocaine "addicts," states that at an earlier period "most of the [cocaine] victims [were] medical men, members of the legal profession, literary men and women, and the cultured generally. We believe at present this type represents only what we may term the sporadic cases, the condition, however being epidemic in the 'tenderloin'."[13] But one must doubt this conclusion. Not only does it fly in the face of historical probability, it is unsupported by any evidence. Nothing in the report so much as implies that either the two authors or other members of the staff had treated upper-class cocaine users prior to 1914, and thus the lack of such admissions between 1914 and 1916 is irrelevant to the question at hand. Moreover, then as now, "a significant number of persons in the higher socioeconomic classes regularly receive drugs without detection or apprehension by enforcement agencies."[14] And the author might have added, without detection by hospital authorities. Only a very small percentage of cocaine users ever overindulge to the point of requiring medical treatment,[15]

103

and the well-to-do user who did do so would hardly apply to a public hospital after the Harrison Act had made it dangerous to reveal one's status as a drug user—not when he could afford to go to his discreet family doctor.

Whatever may be probable, however, there is little hard evidence to show precisely who used cocaine during the first few years after Harrison. Doctors could still prescribe it without being too harassed by the authorities, so one can assume that most of them did prescribe it for those who could pay their fees. And since prohibition always makes drug-selling a profitable enterprise, we know that dealers moved in to supply those who wanted cocaine and couldn't get it elsewhere: "The drug evil has not been lessened in this city [New York] in the opinion of Judge Cornelius F. Collins. . . . He said the profit from selling drugs was so great that criminals went into business. . . . One youth who had come before Collins said 'he could always get narcotics easily whenever he had the money'."[16] Or, nothing changes.

The situation had changed in one respect by the 1920s, however. By that time, law enforcement harassment of doctors had made it difficult to get prescriptions for cocaine and the opiates, and most upper-class users had to buy their supplies from dealers or disreputable druggists just like their less affluent fellow users. As usual, those with money got a better deal. As Dr. Royal S. Copeland, Health Commissioner for New York City, pointed out in 1919, "The rich have the advantage in that they can buy in quantity while the poor are robbed by vendors who charge high prices and adulterate the drug."[17] Dr. Copeland knew what he was talking about. In New York, after the passage of the Smith Anti-Cocaine Bill in 1907, while legal cocaine sold for $2.50 an ounce, or approximately 10 cents a gram, druggists were selling illicit cocaine for $1.00 per one-sixteenth ounce, or about 57 cents a gram, and street dealers were getting 10 cents a blow, or about $5.00 a gram.[18] Put another way, if you were a respectable citizen whom the druggist felt he could trust, you paid five or six times as much as you had the year before, whereas if you were one of the riffraff who had to resort to street dealers, you might be paying fifty times as much. Of course, if you could afford to buy ounces, the price jump wasn't quite so bad. The illicit drug business is like any other, and the customer who buys in quantity gets a better deal. The druggist who charged $1.00 for a sixteenth undoubtedly would sell an ounce for $10. And the street dealer who charged 10 cents a blow wouldn't charge a gram buyer $5.00. (Given the current prices of cocaine—$1,800-$2,000 for a relatively pure ounce—it doesn't appear as if these old coke-heads were undergoing any undue hardships. But things are relative and imagine how it would be if cocaine suddenly jumped to the $6,000 or $8,000 per ounce range, the rate of increase they experienced back in 1907.)

By the 1920s illicit cocaine had risen to $30 an ounce, or three times what it had been a decade earlier.[19] And naturally some people paid considerably more than the acknowledged market price. Tallulah Bankhead's biographer has her paying $50 in the early 1920s to "the urchins who hung around . . . . in the west Forties" for a bag of coke the size of a tea bag.[20] The urchins must have known they had a live one. A tea bag will comfortably hold about four grams of cocaine. If packed to bursting it might accommodate almost twice this much, but dealers have never been known for their generosity. At any rate, when you consider it takes 28 grams to make an ounce, it is clear that Miss Bankhead paid considerably more than the prevailing rate for that which she called "absolutely divine."

According to at least one writer and the recollection of several people who were active during the period, cocaine was common among the high-life set of the twenties. The writer claims that "cocaine . . . was as au courant as marijuana is today [1973].[21] But none of those to whom I talked remembered it as quite that popular. The seemingly most accurate recol-

lection came from a man who had been a member
of some of the well-known bands of the era:

"From what I saw, what you say that fellow
wrote isn't right. I've got a son, a business man
who does pretty well, and he tells me marijuana
is so much around the people he knows that no
one even talks about it. Now a few years ago he'd
tell me about how if someone lit up, these same
people you see, there'd be a whole ceremony, and
a lot of people might take their first tokes and
laugh and giggle a lot and say things like 'Am I
high?'. Now *that's* kind of the way it was with coke,
generally speaking. We'd sometimes play at a party
and the host or hostess would break out some coke,
maybe a half-ounce or an ounce. Just about every-
body would take some, but no two ways about it,
a lot of those people had never seen it before. You'd
have to tell most of the ladies, 'No, you gotta *snort*
it up, not *sniff* it up!' They'd be so dainty about it,
you see. And they were young people, in their
twenties and thirties. You see? If coke was that
much around they'd have known about it better
than they did. I came across more than one *real*
coke group, I can tell you that. Mostly though,
that was musicians. But when something's around
that makes you feel good, you just know there's
going to be more than *one* kind of group doing
what comes naturally. You just know that. I heard
lots of stories but I didn't see it myself except with
the musicians. And except uptown. I had a friend
in the band, a colored fellow, excuse me, black
fellow. Well, he lived up on Lexington, round 128th,
and we were real friends. Lots of times I'd sleep
over at his place, and his wife would make us
breakfast and all. Well, he told me a lot about
Harlem and showed me a lot. We'd all go places,
night clubs, parties, and so on. The point is there
was lots of coke up there, a lot more than downtown. Only it was never as good. It's really true
what they say, the black people get cheated. My

friend told me he never could get coke in Harlem as good as he got downtown. He said lots of times he'd bring some back from some party he'd played at and his friends would think it was too *strong*. They weren't used to it you see. Can you imagine that?"[22]

One can easily imagine it. I have already made the point, and will undoubtedly continue to make it, that the illicit drug business *is* a business essentially like any other; and the factors which lead to ghetto blacks paying more for inferior food than do whites for quality food operate in the illicit drug business too. Cocaine in Harlem is usually heavily adulterated and the Harlem buyer ends up paying considerably more for his cocaine than does the midtown buyer.[23] And this is an old story. In 1901, an officer of the American Pharmaceutical Association noted that the cocaine available to Atlanta blacks was only 25 per cent pure and patronizingly explained that "the darkies seemed to be very well satisfied with that kind of cocaine."[24]

The recollections of people active during the twenties indicate that cocaine use was about as prevalent among the affluent high-rollers as was marijuana among upper middle-class adults in 1970-1971, the years immediately before marijuana became too common to elicit comment. There is no accurate way of estimating either how many people used cocaine or how much of it was used, though we do know that in one way or another considerably more cocaine was available to Americans *after* the Harrison Act was passed than before. And it seems reasonable to suppose that the conscious pleasure use of cocaine increased as well. (In the legal era much of the cocaine was sold and used in the quasi-medical form of tonics, hay fever remedies, cold cures, and the like, and users could easily convince themselves they were taking it not for pleasure but for "legitimate" purposes—as now many dieters who take amphetamines and nervous persons who take tranquilizers convince themselves they use their drugs purely for medical reasons.) The desire for pleasure not being confined to those who can best afford it, the straightforward pleasure use of cocaine had undoubtedly increased all across the economic spectrum, despite a very sharp increase in prices. What little evidence there is, supports this assumption. In 1914 according to Dr. Jackson R. Campbell of the New York City Department of Correction, "Forty per cent of those now confined in the Tombs are habitual users of cocaine."[25] By 1925, some 60 per cent of those committed to the workhouse of Welfare Island were drug users and most of them used cocaine.[26] Since almost no one of means ever got sent to the Welfare Island workhouse, it is safe to assume that these cocaine users were representatives of the economically disadvantaged.

The point is that as with all prohibitions, whether against alcohol, heroin, or homosexuality, the prohibition against cocaine did not work. Those who liked it didn't stop using it any more than did the typical drinker after the passage of the Volstead Act. The prohibition made cocaine more expensive—all black market commodities are more expensive—and eventually the poorest users had to forego it altogether, leaving only the well-to-do as regular users. This was very unlike the situation with the banned opiates. The poor, despite the outrageous prices, never stopped regular use.[27] The reason for this marked difference is, of course, that the opiates are addictive drugs and cocaine is not. The opiate addict undergoing the pains of withdrawal is in no position to ask himself if he can afford relief, he seeks it whatever the cost. The cocaine user, not being in such bondage to his drug, can ask himself if the pleasure is worth the price. If the answer is no, he is not compelled by the needs of his body to pay whatever he must. In short, cocaine users don't steal and mug to raise the price of a gram.

The very fact that the rising cost of cocaine worked to reserve its use to those with money gave it a snob appeal that is still very much with us today. Snorting coke became a sign of knowing sophistication akin to buying suits in London rather than at Brooks Bros.

Survivors of the period attest to this, as does the scanty evidence found in the few literary and musical cocaine references of the time.

The magazine *Vanity Fair*, a publication of such arch and rarified snobbism that the current *Harper's Bazaar* and *New Yorker* seem proletarian in comparison, took note of the 1922 West Coast drug scene in the following words:

"With the brightening influence of spring there has been a distinct quickening of the social pace. Drugs are not as much in evidence as during the more trying days of winter, but they still spread their genial influence at some of the more exclusive functions. Last week little Lulu Lenore of the Cuckoo Comedy Co. gave a small house dance for the younger addicts. 'Will you come to my Snow-Ball?' read the clever invitations. In one corner of the living room was a miniature 'Drug-Store,' where Otho Everard kept the company in a roar as he dispensed little packages of cocaine, morphine, and heroin. The guests at their departure received exquisite hypodermic needles in vanity boxes which have caused many heart-burnings among those who were not invited."[28]

The original lyrics of Cole Porter's "I Get a Kick Out of You" contained the familiar "I get no kick from champagne" but when Mr. Porter, the darling of cafe society, first wrote the song, this verse was followed by:

"I get no kick from cocaine
I'm sure that if
I took even one sniff
It would bore me terrifically too
But I get a kick out of you."

And Charlie Chaplin, in the jail scene in *Modern Times,* snorts a white powdery substance identified as "nose powder" and then, with a great burst of manic energy, proceeds to overpower all obstacles in his path.

(Neither Porter's song nor Chaplin's movie came out in the twenties. "I Get a Kick Out of You" appeared in the 1934 musical *Anything Goes,* and *Modern Times* was first shown in 1936. But I offer them as at least indirect evidence of the twenties cocaine scene rather than that of the thirties on the grounds that (1) *Anything Goes* was set in and reflected the styles of the twenties; and more tenuously (2) though *Modern Times* commented on the first years of the depression, this was a period so close to the roaring twenties that Chaplin could be sure his audience would fully understand the cocaine reference.)

However this may be, the important thing is that highly successful Broadway lyricists don't write songs for the purpose of mystifying the paying customers. When Porter wrote "I get no kick from cocaine . . . but I get a kick out of you," he did so with the perfect assurance that his audience knew the lady in question had made a most powerful impression on him. Similarly, successful magazines are closely geared to the tastes and understanding of their readers. The editors of *Vanity Fair* would never have printed "Happy Days in Hollywood" had they not known that their sophisticated readers would greet it with knowing, appreciative giggles. In both these instances the cocaine reference was designed to titillate the upper-income denizens of the big cities, which was not the case with Chaplin's "nose powder" scene. Movies are made for the mass market and Chaplin's movies, appealing as they did to every sector of society, were enormously successful. And it doesn't seem probable that Chaplin, who was not an artist given to making esoteric in-jokes, would use cocaine as the instigating force of a wildly comic episode unless he was certain that his mass market audience would understand it. The very fact that Chaplin felt able to use such a reference in the mid-thirties, when cocaine had become virtually restricted to the rarified circles of Hollywood and New York, indicates that either it was so widely known to

110

the masses a few years earlier that no one had forgotten it, or that Chaplin believed its prevalence in Hollywood reflected a nationwide pattern. Given his demonstrated acumen concerning his market, this last appears unlikely.

The years of sensational and misleading newspaper and magazine stories linking cocaine with blacks, crime, and depravity may have helped keep cocaine alive in the public consciousness, but they also instilled a deep-seated ambivalence about illicit drugs in general. The public might roar with knowing laughter when the little tramp was transformed into a whirlwind after snorting "nose-powder"—after all *he* would never do it in "real" life—but they had reacted with rage when informed that their idols *did* do such awful things. Public reaction to the Hollywood "dope scandals" of the early twenties prompted the movie industry to create the Hays Office for enforcing a morals code designed to reassure the ticket-buyers that Hollywood was not a haven for degenerates and drug addicts.[29]

The information available on the Hollywood drug scene of the twenties is sensationalistic and about as reliable as your favorite gossip column. Beginning with the Fatty Arbuckle case, the newspapers tried to outdo each other in exposing the "sins" of the movie colony. Arbuckle, a very popular comedian, stood trial on manslaughter charges growing out of the death of a young woman during the course of a party he hosted. The papers carried juicy hints of drugs and sexual perversions in connection with the case but printed nothing explicit about either. By the time they were through, however, Arbuckle had been tried and acquitted three times, and they had inflamed the public's indignation to the point that he never again appeared in a film.[30] Soon after this, the director Desmond Taylor was murdered in his home. Much space was devoted to the theory that Taylor had been done in by a dealer whom he had warned to stop selling drugs to Mabel Normand and other stars at the Mack Sennett Studio.[31] And then in 1922 it was revealed that

111

Wallace Reid, a top screen idol of the day, had been a "drug addict" for the past two years.[32]

The dope scandal stories never reveal *which* drugs the players were using. One old Hollywood hand with whom I have talked said that cocaine was certainly one of the most popular drugs of the era but that morphine and heroin were plentiful too. What little documentary evidence there is, is inferential rather than explicit. Mabel Normand of the Sennett lot, for example, was generally regarded as a cokehead. Sennett's biographer, Gene Fowler, denies this but his denial is damning: "She had sinus trouble, and to alleviate it, she occasionally took a narcotic."[33] The "narcotic" taken for sinus trouble in those days was cocaine. In the Wallace Reid case, though no specific drug is ever mentioned, it seems clear that if his wife is to be believed he too took cocaine:

"Wallace always drank to some extent, and about two years ago began to use drugs. He was very ill at that time but . . . there was a great deal of work at his studio and he felt that he must keep up somehow, so he resorted to artificial means. . . ."[34]

In short, he was using a stimulant which his doctor called a "narcotic" and the newspapers called "dope," but cocaine is the only drug of that time which fits the description.

Because no other country was as afflicted with patent medicines and nostrums, America imported far more coca leaves, made much more cocaine, and was the world's preeminent user from the late nineteenth century to well into the twentieth century—excepting, of course, for the homeland of coca where the Indians chewed it as they always had, and the educated classes used refined cocaine. But cocaine was popular elsewhere, and especially so after World War I. A detailed analysis of foreign use is beyond my power at present, but the few examples I have will at least give some idea of the situation.

112

In India, the cocaine traffic was well organized and extensive: ". . . a large quantity of cocaine is smuggled into the country every year. . . . The provincial excise reports testify to the increase of the cocaine traffic throughout the country. The trade is extremely lucrative. During the war [World War I] the drug sold as high as 450 rupees [$150] an ounce."[35] And by the 1920s, it was estimated that between 250,000 and 500,000 people "were taking cocaine habitually in India for its euphoric effects."[36]

Cocaine was introduced to Egypt around 1918 when, according to a United Nations report, "a Greek chemist domiciled in Cairo succeeded in introducing cocaine into high society and in a few years amassed a colossal fortune."[37] Since it was selling for $75 (Egyptian) per kilogram in the streets of Cairo, he must have been unloading it by the carload to make that much money. If cocaine was so popular in India and Egypt, it is hard to imagine a country where it wasn't doing well.

It certainly made a strong impression on the major capitals of Europe. By the mid-twenties Berlin officials were gravely concerned over the spread of the cocaine habit: "The authorities are . . . in a quandary for a method to suppress the drug at after-theatre parties in private homes, where 'snow' is circulated with the same freedom and nonchalance as cigarettes."[38] Worse yet, "cocaine was said to be most used by the prominent residents of Berlin's fashionable West End and the traffic is especially menacing among the younger artist and actor circles."[39] Such a situation was obviously not to the liking of the narcs, who much prefer busting the less influential types. Fortunately for them, cocaine was used by all classes in Germany: ". . . in the large towns, there are many cocainists in every profession, down to prostitutes and their protectors. . . . In Berlin there are cocaine dens both disreputable and dirty, and also fashionable and up-to-date establishments. One of these was raided at the beginning of the present year [1924]. About one hundred habitués, men and women, from all classes of society,

113

even university and literary men, had gathered there."[40] The going price seems to have been about $5.00 a gram.[41]

The Germans weren't content simply to get high but, if the insinuations of their enemy are to be believed, were determined to recoup some of their war losses by selling cocaine to France. The French repeatedly claimed that most of the cocaine sold in France came from Germany and that Germans brought it in: "Four Germans, two of whom are former officers in the German army, have been arrested as leaders in the biggest plot to smuggle cocaine into France that has come to the attention of the police in many years."[42]

The beneficiaries of this low plot were, as elsewhere in the world, from all classes of society: "Cocaine taking formerly was confined to the habitués of night restaurants in Montmartre and similar resorts . . . it is now common all over Paris, the suburbs, and country."[43] In Paris, cocaine sold for $2.00 to $3.00 a gram and it was usually no more than 25 per cent pure.[44]

Though the French were blaming the Germans for making cocaine readily available in France after the war, this appears to be a typical case of using a popular villain as a scapegoat. There was plenty of cocaine in France *during* the war, when it might be supposed that not much could have been smuggled in from Germany. In "The Nightmare of Cocaine," (By a Former "Snow-Bird"), an American member of the A.E.F. related the following story touching on this point:

"I was honestly frightened many times . . . rain, mud, shells, no relief; literally, Hell. Cognac gone! Spirits lagging! Not exactly frightened but fearful. Oh, for one big drink! But none was there.

"A fellow officer of the French army stood beside me in the rain. His spirits were high, he was happy. I saw him occasionally put a pinch of something in his nostrils, and a moment later his eyes were bright,

114

he was levity in the face of disaster, he was confident. I shuddered—*snow*!

". . . a raid was imminent. Cognac! I fairly prayed for it. I reached out my hand and my companion smiled as he placed in it the tiny box. . . . I took one, two quick sniffs of the snowy powder. There was a momentary burning sensation, quick free breaths, a suffusing warmness, and with it my timidity disappeared. The whining shells became louder—I smiled. A few broke near—I laughed. . . . I patted the shoulder of my French benefactor. . . . He merely shrugged his shoulders, held out the box, and I accepted it once more. . . . Unfortunately cocaine was easy to obtain in France."[45]

And it was common enough that Marcel Proust, who left us the most beautiful and complete account of the disintegration of a social order yet written, made more than passing references to cocaine in his masterpiece, *A La Recherche du Temps Perdu*. In the volume, *The Captive,* published in 1923 but set before the war, he relates how Madame Verdurin

". . . while pretending not to have heard anything, and preserving in her fine eyes, shadowed by the habit of listening to Debussy more than they would have been by that of sniffing cocaine, the extenuated expression that they derived from musical intoxication alone . . . and unable to contain herself any longer, unable to postpone the injection for another instant, flung herself upon the speakers."[46]

And in the last volume, the 1928 *The Past Recaptured,* he touches on the wide social range of cocaine use. In a scene describing the manifold problems and cares attendant to the running of a homosexual bordello during wartime, he quotes the manager, "There's 7 ringing. They say they're sick. Sick my eye! They're coke-fiends. They look half-doped already. I'll have to throw them out."[47] Later in the book he tells us how he

115

"happened to meet in the street, four or five years before, the Vicomtesse de St.-Fiarcie. . . . Her statuesque features seemed to assure her eternal youth. And, besides, she was still young. But now, despite her smiles and greeting, I could not recognize her in a lady whose features were so chipped away that the lines of her face could no longer be reconstructed. What had happened was that she had been taking cocaine and other drugs for three years past. Her eyes, circled with deep black rings, wore almost a haunted look. Her mouth had a peculiar sneer. . . . Time has in this way express trains and special trains to carry people to a premature old age."[48]

Cocaine was equally plentiful in England, and the English, who were so far from being alarmists on the question of habit-forming drugs that they didn't pass a prohibition comparable to our Harrison Act until 1920, and even then left the question of who should be allowed such drugs to the physicians rather than to the police, became so concerned about the rapid spread of cocaine that they passed an anticocaine bill in 1916 which made possession of cocaine by an unauthorized person a felony.[49] And they did this despite the fact the authorities generally agreed that "Prohibition notoriously does not prohibit . . . and the various anti-narcotic laws, including the defective and vexatious Harrison law, merely makes it more difficult and more costly for drug victims to get their favourite narcotic or stimulant."[50]

As it turned out, the authorities should have listened to themselves; for about all this 1916 law did—and all other drug prohibitions then and now—was to increase the price of cocaine and encourage illicit traffic in the drug. Prior to the law, a ten-gram bottle retailed for fifteen shillings; after the law was passed this same bottle sold for from ten to twenty pounds.[51] One well-informed author of the period, Dr. Nathan Mutch, wrote that while it was well known that the

116

use of cocaine was "rife in America and on the Continent" during the 1920s, his countrymen seemed to believe that their anticocaine law had very much reduced such use in England. On the contrary, he said, his analysis of the documented cases of cocaine use and sale between 1920 and 1923 in London revealed that "the practice was for many years rife in London in the post-war period."[52] And if Aleister Crowley's 1922 novel, *Diary of a Drug Fiend,* is to be believed—and it strikes me as both accurate and believable, comparable in these respects to William Burroughs's *Junkie*—it was certainly rife among the English upper classes:

> "We went to tea with Mabel Black. Every one was talking about drugs. Every one seemed to want them; Lord Landsend had just come back from Germany and he said you could buy it [cocaine] quite easily there."[53]

Crowley's great merit in this book is in the aptness of his descriptions. Of the coke-head heroine he writes:

> "Her eyes glittered, her lips twittered, her cheeks glowed like fresh brown buds in spring. She was the spirit of cocaine incarnate; cocaine made flesh."[54]

Of the effects of cocaine:

> ". . . cocaine swept from my nostrils to my brain— the depression lifted from my mind like the sun coming out of the clouds."[55]

> "When one is on one's cocaine honeymoon, one is really, to a certain extent, superior to one's fellows. One attacks every problem with perfect confidence."[56]

> "Used in moderation, we find it to be positively wholesome."[57]

"But cocaine insists upon one's living upon one's capital, and assures one that the fund is inexhaustible."[58]

Of the difficulties of being in a strange city without a connection:

". . . to have to put on a lot of beastly clothes and hunt all around Paris for a dope peddler."[59]

Of what happens when prolonged overindulgence has transformed the effects of the drug:

"We've arranged for a regular supply; but the thing is that the stuff doesn't work any more. We get the insomnia and those things all right, but we can't get any fun out of it."[60]

And of the effect of the 1916 anticocaine law. The speaker is a member of Parliament who just happens to own a cocaine factory on the Continent:

". . . thanks to the very Act which I had so arduously laboured to put upon the statute . . . that little bottle of yours which was sold retail for a matter of fifteen shillings, can now be sold—discreetly, you understand—in the West End for almost anything one cares to ask—ten, twenty, even fifty pounds to the right customer."[61]

And so, to quote a good man once more, it goes.

6

The Great Drought

Though it is not a proposition susceptible to proof, I believe the drugs people use are a fairly reliable barometer of the socioeconomic conditions in which they live, and vice versa. LSD, for example, has never been popular in the black ghettos of America, whereas heroin has always been very popular; and cocaine, the chic drug of the twenties, seems to have virtually disappeared by the thirties. In the first case, LSD, an extremely sensitizing drug, is hardly ideal for watching rats crawl out of walls; while heroin, a central nervous system depressant, might have been designed for such experiences: high on smack, you can watch those rats and not give a damn. In the second case, the twenties was a period of new sexual freedom, easy money, and prevailing optimism—a time well suited to a costly, stimulating euphoric; while by the 1930s the depression had settled in, money was tight, people gloomy, and an expensive "fun" drug like cocaine hardly seemed to fit in. Had it been as cheap as it was a couple of decades earlier, cocaine probably would have held on. People like to get high on their favorite drug no matter how low the national spirits. But recreational drugs are like other recreational materials insofar as people make decisions about their use—and one of the most important questions they ask is, is the high worth the price?

Virtually every source I have consulted agrees that cocaine use was insignificant during the 1930s. Newspapers which had carried many cocaine stories during the twenties carried only very occasional pieces during the thirties. And police officials who had been active in creating the "cocaine menace" for the past twenty years virtually shut up. Instead they issued a steady stream of statements attributing current "crime waves" to marijuana, a drug just beginning to grow in popularity. Despite the obvious differences in the two drugs, these statements read as if the law enforcement spokesmen had simply pulled out their cocaine propaganda file and retyped it, substituting "marijuana" every place "cocaine" appeared. One typical example, coauthored by a member of the Wichita, Kansas, Police Department, flatly stated that the marijuana user was likely to commit "actions of uncontrollable violence, or even murder,"[1] and quoted the chief detective of the Los Angeles Police Department to support this fanciful assertion:

> "In the past we have had officers of this department shot and killed by Marihuana addicts and *have traced the act of murder directly to the influence of Marihuana, with no other motive.* Numerous assaults have been made upon officers and citizens with intent to kill by Marijuana addicts which were directly traceable to the influence of Marihuana."[2]

And the sexual fear aroused by an alien, less-than-lily-white race was blatantly apparent. Good ole boy Harry Anslinger, Commissioner of the Bureau of Narcotics, testifying in favor of the Marihuana Tax

Act of 1937, submitted a communication he had received from the editor of a Colorado newspaper which, after describing an attack by a Mexican-American "under the influence of marijuana" on a girl of the area, went on to say,

"I wish I could show you what a small marijuana cigarette can do to one of our degenerate Spanish-speaking residents. That's why our problem is so great; the greatest percentage of our population is composed of Spanish-speaking persons, most of whom are low mentally, because of social and racial conditions."[3]

Familiar? Well within the lifetimes of the above authors cocaine had been transformed from a wonder drug to an especially dangerous drug by creating a fear among whites that "cocaine-crazed" blacks would run amuck; and here we see the same fear being created about Mexican-Americans and marijuana. Not that the police and other defenders of public virtue esteemed cocaine any more than they had before, but there simply wasn't much of it around. They needed a new menace, and the growing popularity of marijuana conveniently provided one.

Another indication of cocaine's decline can be found in a couple of verses from "Cocaine Habit," a song recorded by the Memphis Jug Band in 1930:

"I went to Mr. Newman's in a lope
Saw a sign on the window said no more dope."

and,

"Since cocaine went out of style
You can catch 'em shooting needles all the while."[4]

More convincingly than anything written by sociologists, narcs, or newspaper reporters, these few lines show how scarce cocaine had become in most parts of the country by 1930. The writers were traveling musicians, fond of coke, and if they couldn't find any there just wasn't much around to be found.

Cocaine had not, of course, entirely disappeared from the American scene. Its reputation as a producer of euphoric highs was too firmly established to be completely extinguished by laws and campaigns against the evils of cocaine. The depression and the high price of cocaine had drastically reduced the number of people using it, but there were still those who wanted and could afford it. Who they were is difficult to say. The evidence is very scanty. Some authorities mention its continuing availability in black ghettos, among jazz musicians and bohemians, and in Hollywood circles, but I have not come across any who cite references for this information. I have, however, spoken to a few people who moved in these circles during the thirties and the consensus of their opinions is that, yes, cocaine was still around, but not *much* around. It was scarce, and rarely seen except among some groups in Hollywood. My Hollywood correspondent reports that though cocaine was not out in the open as it had been during the early twenties, there was still plenty of it around. In his opinion, most of those who had been into coke were still into it—though cautious about revealing their use to anyone outside their immediate circle. "They liked coke," he said. "They had the money, so they didn't have much trouble getting it. They didn't flash it around though, it was strictly on the quiet."[5]

This isn't a very strong historical brew and until some doctoral candidate ferrets out a sizable number of knowledgeable survivors of the 1930s and records their recollections of cocaine use we are not likely to learn much about the situation.

One curious piece of memorabilia I came across does shed some further light on the presence of cocaine in Hollywood during the period: the 1939 movie, *The Cocaine Fiends* directed by Wm. A. O'Connor. Starting with the pious "public service" announcement on the dangers of the "dope traffic" and the great need for "an aroused and educated public" to combat it, *The Cocaine Fiends* appears to be a quintessential antidrug flick. Jane Bradford, a small-town girl from a poor but good family, meets a hoodlum on the lam who attempts to sweet-talk her into accompanying him to the big city. She wants to go but decides she can't leave her widowed mother. The conflict gives her a headache, at which point the hood—whom we have previously encountered in the opening scene, on his way to sell coke to schoolchildren—says here, doll, take a little of this headache powder. Oh, it's marvelous, I feel better already, cries the fair and foolish maiden. He gives her a little more. It works. I feel swell, I'll go with you, she says with a big smile.

Well, after this initial encounter with the dreaded cocaine it's all downhill. Once in the big city, she finds out that the headache powders she has come to rely on are dope! cocaine! And the thug who promised to marry her has something else in mind. He intends to give her to his boss, the dope-king, who has a fondness for pretty young things. She is repelled by it all but she's helpless, hopelessly hooked, a drug addict: I'll do anything, just give me some! The plot thickens—her brother comes to hunt for her, he in turn gets "hooked" by his dope fiend girl friend, and so on. Finally there's a big recognition scene. Both sister and brother have taken to opium and they meet in an opium den: Jane!—There is no Jane anymore. I'm Lil, a gangster's discarded moll. And then . . . but enough. Suffice it to say that cocaine has ruined their lives. The brother may pull through, but Jane knows it's all up with her: It's too late for me, girls can't go home. Eventually the dope king, an eminent businessman and civic leader, is shot by his own daughter who ends up in the loving arms of the narc who has chased him down.

In every obvious aspect *The Cocaine Fiends* is the peer of the marijuana epic, *Reefer Madness,* and other imaginative antidope creations. Like them it is a repository of the traditional clichés: one snort (or puff or shot) and you're hooked; the absolute causal connection between dope and "sin"; and the inevitable fall from respectability to a shameful and hopeless life. But on closer examination, or on reflection, it becomes clear that *The Cocaine Fiends* is not a standard antidrug piece if only because whoever wrote it had firsthand knowledge of cocaine. Several scenes depict various characters snorting coke, and in none of them are there any exaggerated reactions. They're not transformed into manic power freaks; they don't become hysterical or shriek with laughter, they simply begin to feel good and show signs of increased energy. One begins to wonder what's going on. Everything else in the movie perfectly fits the hallowed fantasy that it's so good and/or bad that you'd better not try it even once or *this* is what will happen. (As in if you smoke one cigarette you're going to end up with lung cancer.) Well, not quite everything; there's one other odd thing about *The Cocaine Fiends:* the fact that it was made in 1939. What's curious about this is that there was next to no publicity on cocaine during the 1930s. Plays, books, and movies with drug themes, and now television dramas, almost always appear in response to publicity on drugs, they rarely anticipate it. This is especially the case with the traditional drugs-are-hell theme. And the bigger the audience commanded by the media, the more closely tied to public expectations it is. But if my research and that of everyone who has written on the subject is correct, cocaine was certainly not a subject on the public's mind in 1939. Why then produce a grade B cocaine movie? Well either all the researchers are dead wrong and cocaine *was* a big issue in 1939, or the movie was conceived a decade earlier but got delayed, or those responsible were coke-heads doing a spoof on the drug-movie genre. The last possibility best explains the picture's curious combination of realism and fantasy. For the makers, like all put-on artists, wanted to be sure that the knowing would catch the spoof; and what better way could they show us they understood cocaine than by showing us they understood its effects?

124

At any rate, the distinction of being the world's biggest user of cocaine had, in the 1930s, passed from America to Germany, which under the Nazis was having something of an economic revival.[6] But apart from the fact that Field Marshal Hermann Göring used cocaine for many years and that Hitler once called him a drug addict;[7] the fact that Hitler often behaved like someone on cocaine or speed;[8] statements and observations to the effect that Hitler was taking stimulants ("As time went on, Morell, his drug doctor, naturally had to resort to stronger drugs and shorter intervals in order to maintain Hitler's performance"; He was incessantly taking some drug or other;"[9] "In the euphorias produced by his drugs he seemed to glow like a wraith."[10]); and general rumors that the Nazi hierarchy harbored more than a few coke-heads, I have found very little material on the subject of cocaine use in Germany during the 1930s. Admittedly my research in this area was cursory, and a more diligent scholar may unearth some interesting material. At any rate the bulk of this chapter and the rest of the book will only occasionally stray from the American scene.

Apart from the changed economic conditions which put cocaine out of the reach of most Americans, its decline in popularity was hastened by another factor: the introduction in 1932 of the amphetamines.[11] The new drug was manna from heaven for all those who because of the expense and scarcity of cocaine were doing without the stimulants they wanted. The amphetamines were legal, readily available, and exceedingly cheap. For a tiny fraction of what it would cost to stay high on cocaine for half an hour, one could, with a single tablet, speed along happily for several hours. Of course the high wasn't really the same. There were *gross* similarities—wakefulness, decreased feelings of fatigue, increased energy, euphoria, and so on—but no connoisseur would ever confuse cocaine with the amphetamines. But most cocaine users were not, and are not, connoisseurs. They were looking for a strong stimulant and the amphetamines were certainly that. When a market exists, something or someone will move in to supply it.

Given their power and cheapness, the incredible growth rate of amphetamine was inevitable. By 1971 eight billion doses of some thirty-one different amphetamines and meta-amphetamine preparations were being legally manufactured by fifteen pharmaceutical houses, to say nothing of the contributions from the illegal speed labs.[12] As diet pills, pep pills, antifatigue pills, antidepressant pills, and simply as get-high pills, amphetamines were and are being used by every class of Americans. There were reports of heavy amphetamine use by businessmen and athletes as early as 1940, and such reports always lag many years behind the phenomena they describe.[13] During WW II armies on both sides issued amphetamines to the troops just as Dr. Aschenbrandt issued cocaine back in 1883. And during the Korean war amphetamines even replaced cocaine in the traditional speedball (cocaine and heroin), the invention apparently of American servicemen stationed in Korea and Japan where both heroin and the amphetamines were cheap and plentiful.[14]

Another striking parallel between the amphetamines and cocaine is that one of the earliest and equally mistaken uses of injected amphetamines was in the treatment of opiate addiction. Several San Francisco physicians took this blind alley in the late 1950s.[15] A few years later the era of the speed freak was in full bloom, a bloom that faded rather quickly as the drug culture woke to the fact that speed was a less than perfect drug. Years of being hassled by crazy, paranoid speed lovers, and seeing their friends wasted by overindulgence, had enlightened the community. No one wanted to be around a speed freak and the popularity of the amphetamines in the world of illicit drug users had declined precipitously by 1968 or 1969. In the straight world of the housewife and the businessman no such rapid decline is evident—diet and pep pills are still very popular. (And from my observa-

126

tions of the street scene, speed seems to be making a comeback—the result, probably, of the current outrageous price of cocaine.)

During this climb of the amphetamines to All-American status cocaine was somewhat in the position of a team that once had known greatness but had lingered in the cellar for many years. It still had its hard-core fans but their number was greatly reduced, and the headlines were few and far between. Occasionally a sign appeared indicating that cocaine was becoming a respectable contender once again—Narc Commissioner Harry Anslinger reported in 1949 "that the U.S. was swamped with the biggest influx of cocaine in 20 years"[16]—but these omens were about as believable as the yearly predictions that the New York Giants football team is a bona fide Super Bowl contender. Anslinger was notorious for his factless hyperbole and his ability to milk the Congress for funds; and, since he had already assured the country that the heroin "menace" was licked, hinting a new cocaine "menace" was just a ploy to keep his budget up.

Nothing of further insignificance on the subject was heard from him until he was appointed U.S. representative to the United Nations Commission on Narcotics in 1962, the year in which the World Health Organization's Expert Committee on Addiction-Producing Drugs, together with the Permanent Central Opium Board of the U.N., began a campaign to persuade the coca-growing nations to eliminate coca-chewing among their Indian populations. As a means, probably, of inducing support for their position from the industrial nations, these U.N. bodies cited the growing incidence of cocaine being smuggled out of the coca-producing countries and into the richer countries, especially the United States.[17] Anslinger, perhaps forgetting his 1949 statement, but more likely remembering the very small number of cocaine busts during the intervening years and not being a man who ever admitted his performance to be less than perfect, assured the United Nations that "cocaine abuse is not at present a problem in the U.S.A."[18] Two years

127

later, however, he appeared willing to accept the proposition that "the situation with respect to cocaine had worsened in recent years."[19]

Perhaps it had, but there is little to support this view other than the fact that in December of 1964 the Bureau of Customs announced "the largest shipment of cocaine ever seized in this country."[20] The shipment weighed in at 22 pounds, and the Bureau's grand total for the fiscal year 1964 came to 28 pounds.[21] Not very much compared to the 619 pounds seized in 1972, when speed was no longer an important factor in the illicit drug scene and cocaine was booming.[22]

The various government agencies responsible for stemming the flow of drugs into the country have conspicuously failed in this impossible task, but insofar as it is reasonable to assume that the more drugs that come in, the more they are likely to seize, the record of their annual seizures does serve as a rough indicator of what is happening on the drug scene. Here then is a listing of cocaine seizures by the Bureau of Customs between 1960 and 1972.[23]

1960	11	pounds
1961	8	"
1962	19	"
1963	10	"
1964	28	"
1965	37	"
1966	45	"
1967	40	"
1968	98	"
1969	199	"
1970	227	"
1971	408	"
1972	619	"

These figures in no way serve as a barometer of the total quantity of cocaine entering the country—the "rule of thumb" which assumes that the drugs seized represent 10 per cent of the total flow is without basis either in theory or fact—but they do, beginning around 1968, reflect the reemergence of cocaine as a popular drug, a fact attested to by users, by law enforcement people, and by medical personnel.

In a 1971 press conference, John Finlator, the then Deputy Director of the Bureau of Narcotics and Dangerous Drugs, stated that "We are finding more of it [cocaine] on the street . . . as recently as three years ago there was little or none of it."[24] On the same day *The New York Times* reported, "Government officials and others say the re-emergence of cocaine is one of the few clear trends in the shifting and often murky picture of drug use in the United States"; also that correspondents from nine of the eleven major college campuses sampled "reported that cocaine use is on the rise"; and that Dr. David Smith, director of San Francisco's Haight-Ashbury Free Medical Clinic, said that in 1971 the use of cocaine had increased more than that of any other drug.[25]

In 1969, when cocaine was half the price it is now, a survey of Dallas schoolchildren revealed that 5 per cent of 7,483 twelfth-graders had used cocaine at least once, in contrast to 17 per cent who had used marijuana at least once.[26] And a 1969 study of 781 Madison, Wisconsin, high school students showed that 5.6 per cent had tried cocaine and that 2.2 per cent used it "frequently," compared to 22.6 per cent who had tried marijuana and 5.1 per cent who used it frequently.[27] On a larger scale, a 1970 assessment of drug use in the general population of New York State concluded that 2.8 per cent (approximately 373,000 persons) of all those fourteen years of age and older had used cocaine at least once and that some 101,000 persons had used cocaine not more than six times per month between March and August of 1970.[28]

The Haight-Ashbury Free Clinic published a study showing an increasing use of cocaine among heroin users. Of 303 seen between March 1971 and September 1971, 10 per cent reported moderate to heavy use of cocaine over the past two months; of 264 seen between September 1971 and January 1972, 13.6 per cent reported the same; and between February 1972 and April 1972, 20.7 per cent of 147 heroin users reported moderate to heavy use of cocaine.[29]

In the same vein a 1973 report revealed that 17.5 per cent of a sample taken from New York City methadone patients were using cocaine.[30]

At best, these figures indicate a trend of increasing cocaine use over the past few years. They in no way indicate the true prevalence of cocaine in our culture. This is not the fault of the researchers; rather it is a difficulty inherent in the very nature of the subject matter. Using illicit drugs is a crime and to expect accurate figures of such use would be as foolish as expecting a Mafia accountant to publish figures which accurately reflected the true sources of his employer's income. The actual numbers of cocaine users cannot, therefore, be established. All we really can determine is that cocaine use in America has been increasing rapidly.

A further, and to my mind more convincing, indication of the rebirth of cocaine is the increasing reference to it in the popular arts and mass media from the late 1960s to the present. Before looking at a sampling of these references, however, it seems worthwhile to spend a little time considering why they are of particular significance.

I began this book by noting the obvious fact that the human race has taken to heart the biblical injunction to use the fruits of the earth for the benefit of mankind, to the degree at least that we have always used whatever substances were available to alter our consciousness. Different societies have used different drugs, but none has long remained content to forego the use of anything likely to relieve in one way or another the stresses of civilization. This being a fact of our universal history one might reasonably expect to find the drug preferences and the effects of these preferences on a particular culture reflected in the standard histories. But this is not the case. A student may be exposed to the most extensive formal education our society can offer and, with the exception of

130

the political ramifications of the prohibition on alcohol, learn nothing about this basic factor of civilization. (For the past several years schoolchildren have been exposed to "drug education" classes; but these are education in only the propaganda sense. They are designed to enforce the establishment's fear of drugs, not to educate the students on the role of drugs in the culture.)

Apart from the reluctance of any establishment to countenance the dissemination of objective information concerning the substances which the people it controls use to escape the pressures of the society, the chief reason for this neglect may be found in the difficulties inherent in writing the history of any thing or any time. The sheer overwhelming numbers of events, the problems of adequately documenting them, and the difficulty of properly interpreting them, necessitate exceedingly condensed accounts. For these reasons, plus the typical historian's fascination with great men and great events, history is rarely more than the bare outlines of how the leading figures or ruling classes of a society responded to the traumas of an era: war, pestilence, and economic dislocation. Revisionist historians such as the Marxists reject such interpretations of events and seek to expose the underlying causes. They seldom, however, mention drugs unless to show the inadequacies of an economic system which gives rise to the use of such products.[31]

There are a few exceptions to this indictment, a handful of historians or investigators who have taken careful note of the role of drugs in a given society: Henry Julian Hunter, *Report of the Medical Officer of the Privy Council* (England, 1864); Terry and Pellens, *The Opium Problem* (America, 1924); Alfred Lindesmith, *The Addict and The Law* (America, 1965); Edward Brecher, *Licit & Illicit Drugs* (America, 1972); Richard Ashley, *Heroin* (America, 1972); and David Musto, *The American Disease* (America, 1973). But all of these, plus a few I haven't listed, are relatively specialized studies and do not receive wide circulation. There has, of course, been a flood of drug books in recent years but almost all of them fall into one of three categories: personal confessions of a drug user; hortatory essays on the evils of drugs; and studies of drug users as members of a "deviant subculture." Except by implication, you will not learn from these that drugs are part of the fabric of society; you will learn, rather, that drugs are a "problem" either to be suppressed by force or eliminated by adequate "education."

It is hard to know what is really going on in your own era; it is harder yet to reconstruct the past; and attempting to do so on the basis of thoroughly inadequate records is a nightmare. The lack, therefore of adequate scholarly attention to drugs makes a difficult task far more difficult than it would otherwise be. This is especially true when the role of a specific drug is in question. And when the drug is one that has not been accepted by the mass of people as, say, alcohol has been, the difficulties are particularly acute. Such is the case with cocaine.

Fortunately, there does exist a body of material which sheds further light on the role cocaine has played in Western culture. It is not extensive, but its very existence indicates that cocaine had a far greater impact than one could gather from any standard history or from any typical drug book. I refer here to the way in which cocaine has been portrayed in novels, plays, movies, and songs, and commented on by pop journalists. (And in television, of course, but the few references I have seen are too recent to be included. I do recall some coke talk on one of the *Kojak* episodes.) I have previously noted that popular artists aren't in the habit of using references not likely to be understood by their audiences. And from this premise I draw the general rule that to the degree a specific illicit drug is celebrated in the popular arts of a period, the drug is accepted in that period; and as an obvious corollary, that the degree of acceptance of a specific drug is further reflected by the degree of attention it receives from those who write about drugs. So far as I am aware, these rules do not apply when

132

a drug is chiefly used under the cloak of medication or when a prescribed drug is used for purposes other than the intent of the prescription. To be sure when the recreational use of prescribed drugs becomes notorious—as in the case of the barbiturates and amphetamines—comments are made. For example, the biggest selling novel of the sixties, *Valley of the Dolls,* celebrated the use of such drugs in Hollywood. Indeed the term "dolls," as slang for them, was coined by the author in the apparent hope of giving her title the resonance provided by a double-meaning. New language, however, is not created by writers of Ms. Susann's abilities, and "dolls" never became an accepted drug term.

There are very few mentions of cocaine in any form from 1930 through 1968, and most of the examples which follow appeared between 1969 and 1974. But reality is not constituted for the convenience of authors. Many cocaine-using musicians either weren't interested or didn't take the trouble to write a coke song. Similarly many cocaine-using authors haven't directly incorporated their drug experiences into their work. Baudelaire, for example, wrote nothing on the subject; nor did Herbert Spencer mention his use of morphine. Then too there are always those who anticipate a trend and cannot be fitted into a convenient time scheme. The most notable examples respecting cocaine are David Musto's 1968 "A Study in Cocaine, Sherlock Holmes and Sigmund Freud"[32] and two songs by Laura Nyro—her 1966 "Buy and Sell" (Cocaine and quiet beers/Sweet candy and caramel/pass the time and dry the tears/on a street called buy and sell), and her 1967 "Poverty Train" (Now/I swear there's something better than/getting off on sweet cocaine/it feels so good/it feels so good/getting off the poverty train/mornin).

But these are anticipatory flashes of a recognition which became more widespread in 1969. Laura Nyro was still a minor cult figure in 1966 and 1967, and Musto's essay appeared in the staid pages of the

Journal of the American Medical Association. Johnny Cash, however, was a major country and western star and his "Cocaine Blues" (Lay off that whiskey and let that cocaine be) came out in 1969. As did, far more significantly, Dennis Hopper and Peter Fonda's film *Easy Rider*—whose heroes not only finance their escape from the workaday world by selling a sizable quantity of cocaine to a customer who arrives for the exchange in a chauffeur-driven Rolls, but who themselves snort it, smoke grass, and drop acid. (The buyer was played by Phil Spector who in real life was to later send a Christmas card to his friends bearing the inscription "A Little 'Snow' At Christmas Time Never Hurt Anyone.") The audiences of *Easy Rider* were neither mystified nor turned off by all this drug-taking: the film became an enormous success, outgrossing such spectaculars as *Lawrence of Arabia* and *A Man for All Seasons.*[33]

In 1970 there was to my knowledge only one film that mentioned cocaine—Billy Wilder's *The Private Life of Sherlock Holmes,* but three songs by major rock groups got into coke: The Rolling Stones' "Let It Bleed" (And there will always be a space in my parking lot/when you need a little coke and sympathy); the Grateful Dead's "Casey Jones" (Driving that train/High on cocaine/Casey Jones you'd better/Watch your speed) which begins with a loud and professional snort; and the Dead's "Trucking" (Living on reds, vitamin C, and cocaine).

(Some officious hypocrites[34] became so incensed by the mention of illicit drugs in rock songs that the FCC was moved to threaten the licenses of any station that played them. A sterling example of the ostrich syndrome, or, put your head in the sand and those nasty people will go away. But to either blame or congratulate the groups who sang about cocaine for its rise in popularity is ludicrous. They didn't import it, they didn't sell it, they simply used it and sang about it. It is equally true, however, that cocaine really took off in 1970 and that rock stars are stylesetters for their fans. When they start using a drug or wearing platform shoes, a lot of people follow suit.)

By 1971 there was no question but that cocaine was firmly reestablished in America. Folk musicians Fred Neil and Hoyt Axton both composed cocaine songs. Neil's "Sweet Cocaine" was a rework of the old "Cocaine Blues," and Axton's "Snow Blind Friend" (Did you say you saw your friend flying low/Dying slow . . . Blinded by snow) sung by Steppenwolf, lamented a buddy who had gotten too deep into cocaine. Rock was represented by the Stones' "Sister Morphine" (Sweet cousin cocaine laid his cool, cool hands on my head) and two songs from Jefferson Airplane personnel: "Mau Mau" (Calling for acid, cocaine, and grass/And receiving your homemade gin) and "Earth Mother" (Earth Mother children here/ripped on coke and feeling dandy). More significantly perhaps, the establishment awoke to cocaine's new status. The *JAMA* printed Dr. Myron Schultz's "The Strange Case of Robert Louis Stevenson" which I have described in Chapter 3. *Newsweek,* under the heading "It's the Real Thing" in its Life and Leisure section, reported that "Evidence of coke's increasing popularity is abundant," and went on to detail how chic coke had become among upper middle-class grass smokers and affluent business and professional types. They ended this rundown by citing one lawyer who "leaves snuff boxes and drinking straws around his house as casual evidence of his new interest."[35]

Rolling Stone, the bible of the pop-rock culture, carried "Cocaine: A Flash In The Pan, A Pain In The Nose" by Jerry Hopkins who ominously noted that the new "in" drug was already "responsible for wasting a number of top musical names and is popular enough to create a new industry: cocaine paraphernalia." When Hopkins gets down to cases his "number of top musical names" wasted by coke becomes one wasted musician who goes nameless, and all in all his piece is largely an up-to-date version of the perennial favorite, the menace of cocaine: "I don't say pure coke *will* kill you, but there's a great possibility."[36]

Which, since there hasn't been a death recorded from the recreational use of coke in at least forty years,[37] goes somewhat beyond the limits of exaggeration permitted even sensationalist writers. What is important about the Hopkins piece, though, is that *Rolling Stone* saw fit to run it as a page one, lead story—something they would not have done if cocaine had not made a great impact on the scenes they observe. More indicative yet of cocaine's new position was the appearance in *Esquire* and *New York* magazines of prepublication selections from Richard Woodley's book, *Dealer, Portrait of a Cocaine Merchant,* a first-rate, authentic profile of a small-time Harlem coke dealer.[38] When good writers do books on a new scene, and major magazines publish excerpts from them, you can rest assured something is going on.

From 1969 through 1971, then, there is an apparent pattern of increasing recognition of cocaine. More rock groups do songs with coke references, more magazines do articles on cocaine, and a serious, accurate study of one facet of the coke culture appears. All of this reflected a marked and progressive increase in the number of people using cocaine.

By 1972 when, as most observers agree, cocaine use continued to grow but at a slower rate than the preceding two years because the expansion had made it available to most of those who wanted to try it, certain noticeable changes occurred in the way cocaine was presented to the public. For one thing no major rock group issued a coke song, at least not to my knowledge. Either it had been around long enough that it was no longer a novelty, or the increasing attention paid it by narcs had made it judicious to be circumspect. (Curtis Mayfield on the other hand recorded no less than four songs which mentioned the drug, the hit, "Superfly," being one of them.) *Newsweek* ran an article on cocaine smuggling which reflected law enforcement's increased concern with the stimulant.[39] *Rolling Stone* published an historical study written in a far more matter of fact tone than the piece of the previous year.[40]

And a little white book appeared, courtesy of the White Mountain Press, which offered the buyer "a complete guide to cocaine."[41] Though not a complete guide and not free from error, it provided the average coke user all the practical information he was likely to need—on dealing practices, weights, prices, cuts, and so on. Selected booksellers in Los Angeles, San Francisco, and New York have said they couldn't keep the book in stock. Knowing members of the fraternity weren't surprised, but their straighter colleagues were amazed that a small book—its contents would fill no more than thirty pages of a standard-sized trade book—with a price tag of $5.00 kept selling out as fast as they got it in. A lot of people wanted basic user information, which would hardly have been the case if a lot of people weren't using cocaine.

But for the historian of cocaine the most important publishing event of 1972 was the appearance in *Esquire* of work-in-progress by Bruce Jay Friedman, later published as Section 4, "Lady," in his 1974 novel *About Harry Towns*. Lady, an affectionate term for cocaine, depicts the late sixties or early seventies Manhattan coke scene as experienced by an affluent screen writer. No one who knew that scene can doubt that Friedman knew it too, but what is important is that he chose to write about it and become the first popular novelist since Conan Doyle and, stretching the category, Aleister Crowley, to make cocaine a major factor in the life of his protagonist. And unlike either of his predecessors he doesn't sensationalize the subject.

Friedman begins the Lady section by telling us what coke means to his hero: "If Harry Towns had a slim silver foil packet of it against his thigh—which he did two or three nights a week—he felt rich and fortified, almost as though he were carrying a gun."[42] Then, his growing disenchantment with the constant search for coke, which is the lot of the gram buyer, leads Harry to become an ounce buyer. For a moment he tries to tell himself that now he has a lot of it and doesn't have to keep looking for more, he won't

137

use as much. "But he got on to himself in a second and knew it wasn't going to work out that way. He'd take more."[43] And Harry does take more, but Friedman doesn't stoop to any nonsense about how poor old Harry disintegrates under the impact of all that coke. No, Harry is representative of his kind and though his lifestyle becomes more centered around the use of cocaine, he isn't led into incredible excesses, he doesn't end up in Bellevue, and he isn't transformed into a brutal, aggressive coke fiend. Rather coke changes the order of his life just as any shiny, new, much-wanted toy changes a person's life. The Triumph owner who gets a Ferrari drives it more than he did his old car—for a while anyway. And this is what happens to the small-bore coke user who suddenly has all the coke he wants. In both cases the novelty of having all you want of what you want fades after a while, and one gets back to facing life on more realistic terms. Sometimes this happens as a matter of course, the bloom fading with the passage of time. And sometimes it happens in response to a new awareness: that driving that fast can get you killed, or that using that much coke puts a strain on your resources—financial, emotional, and physical—you don't really want or need. One way or another, it happens. Unless of course you happen to be one of the very few who either lacks or fails to use his common sense. Harry Towns had the sense to realize he had been overdoing the coke, and so do most users when and if they are ever in such a position.

Why, though, should a serious novelist's realistic depiction of one slice of a coke-head's life be regarded as an event that tells us much about cocaine's place in the culture? Well for one thing, Friedman treats Harry Towns's use of cocaine as simply a part, if an important part, of Harry's life. It leads him into new adventures but they are not adventures at odds with his character. Nothing happens which jars the reader into a "What, Harry Towns doing that?" response. Cocaine is treated, in short, as an adjunct to Harry's life, not as a prime moving force. Which is the way things really are with coke. The other thing is that Friedman uses cocaine as a novelistic device in the way other writers have used, say, alcohol or money. That is, as a tool for both defining a character's milieu and revealing his manner of dealing with himself and others. And no serious novelist would use cocaine for these purposes unless he was reasonably certain that his readers would not be so stunned by its exotic nature that they would be distracted from following the development of the leading character.

Friedman apparently felt this certainty, and he was right. For by 1972 cocaine was no novelty, and especially not to the affluent types who had been smoking marijuana for a few years. These people, for whom grass had replaced the predinner martini and other like pastimes, were buyers in the illicit drug market and naturally met up with cocaine. They are garment district executives, models, designers, salesmen, admen, doctors, lawyers, bankers, professors, writers—indeed they simply represented a healthy cross-section of those who lead the good life in America's major cities. And just as at an earlier time they had been introduced to marijuana by a friend, they were now introduced to cocaine. Marijuana hadn't hurt them so they saw no good reason not to try cocaine. Moreover the police and the media had given it such an incredible reputation that it would hardly have been human not to give it a try. As things turned out it was nowhere near so outrageous as they had been led to believe, but it did make them feel good, and they rarely noticed any bad aftereffects. Of course it was very expensive and not so easy to get as grass. Consequently, few of them used cocaine with anything like the regularity they used marijuana. They reserved it for special occasions, much as they would an expensive wine. Only a miniscule percentage ever got into coke on the Harry Towns level. Equally few of them had ever gotten to the point where they regularly sat around day after day stoned out on marijuana, and now they didn't get high night after night on cocaine. They found that a moderate use of cocaine didn't seem to have any adverse effects, and they liked it that way.

There's not an awful lot to say about cocaine and the media in 1973. By this time it was so well entrenched and so important an item in the drug culture that *The New York Times* carried more stories on coke busts than on heroin busts. And so established that, given the pace of the rock world, writing a song about it may have seemed anachronistic: Doug Sahm's "Dealer's Blues" (Well you need a lotta cocaine/to get a lotta rhythm and blues) being the only such 1973 song I know of. Cocaine's status in the chic set was also acknowledged, though somewhat belatedly, by *New York* magazine which felt compelled to announce it was *the* drug.[44] And its place in the public consciousness was such that the hugely successful movie *Superfly* had as its hero a cocaine dealer who not only defeats the crooked narcs but lives happily ever after on his coke profits. Indeed cocaine had reached the stage where the Drug Enforcement Administration (successor to the Bureau of Narcotics and Dangerous Drugs which had succeeded the Federal Bureau of Narcotics —or DEA out of BNDD out of FBN, a three-horse parlay that has made a lot of dealers rich) was devoting 50 per cent of its effort to combating the traffic in cocaine.[45]

I really shouldn't do what I am about to do, namely, take note of and criticize a book whose only discernible value escapes me, but there *is* a reason. Or, rather, there are two reasons. To state them briefly, when law enforcement agencies cooperate with allegedly independent writers in the production of rank antidrug propaganda on a specific drug there is (a) about as definitive proof as you can desire that the drug in question is very big, and (b) on occasion such trash should be exposed for what it is.

The trash I refer to is a 1973 paperback original by one Marc Olden, which from information largely supplied by federal narcotics officers purports to tell "all" about the New York coke scene. What the unfortunate buyer of this little book got was not a portrayal of using and dealing in the big city, but a tacky farrago of fantasies, an unlikely proportion of which centered on the sexual games supposedly played by Cuban dealers and their women—games which only the participants or voyeurs could describe, neither of which roles is claimed by the author or his narc informants. But this is only the hot sauce; the "hard" information is considerably more unbelievable. For apart from several anecdotes showing dealers doing business in ways so unprofessional and foolish that if this were standard operating procedure the only cocaine available would be that sold by the police, the book is filled with such meretricious gems as:

"It's possible to get a habit just from handling the drug."[46] (Absolutely untrue.)

"Cocaine dealers think along lines that are often hard to understand. Several say they're dealing cocaine because if caught, the jail sentence is less than for heroin."[47] (No coke dealer I ever knew or heard of was ignorant of the drug laws.)

"Narcs say that whores are deep into coke. 'All of 'em, all of 'em,' says Joe. . . . Few are into heroin . . . it's deteriorating."[48] (Heroin is the most common drug used by prostitutes. Indeed a good percentage of them become prostitutes in order to support their habits.)

"Junkies use coke, among other things, as a substitute for heroin."[49] (Totally false. Cocaine is a CNS stimulant, heroin a CNS depressant. They have opposite effects and one *cannot* be the substitute for the other. To belabor the point: if coke was a substitute for heroin, an addict could stave off the pains of withdrawal with cocaine, as he can with methadone. But he can't.)

To believe any of the above quotations requires, as does any single page of the book, a total ignorance of cocaine and the drug world. Its sole importance lies in the fact that federal narcotics officers saw fit to vent either their fantasies or their propaganda in such a shoddy production. And I can think of no clearer sign than this to indicate the importance cocaine has assumed in the drug market.

The situation changed in many ways after 1972, and most of the changes resulted from cocaine's continued and increasing popularity The next chapter discusses these changes and everything else relevant to the current situation—prices, dealing practices, and so on. But in concluding this chapter it is worth noting that the United States Congress, a body not known for responding to changed conditions until they are too obvious to ignore, devoted the major part of a 1973 report on the world drug situation to the cocaine traffic emanating from Latin America. The report's introduction contains the following appraisal: "Firm statistics are not available on the number of cocaine users in the United States, although the number is believed to be both substantial and growing."[50]

One further sign of cocaine's solid position in the drug culture was the appearance in 1974 of two serious studies of the drug: *Cocaine Papers* (New York, Stonehill Publishing Co.), a new translation of Freud's five papers, with commentaries by several writers; and the book you are now reading. Neither could have found a trade publisher a few years ago; interest in the subject simply not being widespread enough. It is now, and in the near future the market will be flooded with books on cocaine.

7

Caveat Emptor, or The Way Things Are Now and Methods of Testing Cocaine

The return of the native after an absence of several centuries is a stock plot in science fiction. Nothing is familiar, everything has changed. Had a New York coke-user been away from the city between 1971 and 1973, a mere two years or so, he might feel equally ill at ease and out of place when he returned. When he left a pure gram of Bolivian flake, the best illicit cocaine available, could be had for from $40 to $50, and it wasn't especially hard to find; a quarter-ounce (7 grams) went for $200-225; and an ounce brought $600-700. By 1972 pure grams of fine coke could still be had if your connections were good, but they were selling for $60-75 and an uncut ounce cost $800-1,000. The casual small buyer, however, was not likely to score pure coke. The situation got much worse in 1973. Even the dealer couldn't get pure cocaine unless he were large enough to buy in kilos, and the small buyer hadn't a chance of getting a pure gram unless the dealer was a personal friend. Pure ounces were going from $1,200 to $1,500 when they were available, and they weren't usually available. By 1974 things had gotten to the point where good cocaine was as hard to find in New York as an honest narc. When a pure ounce of good cocaine was on the market the asking price was $1,800-2,000 and the dealer who two years before provided an ounce customer with a free "tasting" gram as a matter of course, now demanded $90 for it. There was cheaper coke. The Cuban dealers were much into selling 20-25 per cent coke at $500-600 an ounce, but this was cocaine like commercial white bread is bread—with most of the essential ingredients processed out.

Many things contributed to this turn of events in New York. The narcs like to point to the stringent new law that went into effect September 1, 1973, a Draconian measure which made life sentences without parole a distinct possibility for anyone convicted of selling "narcotics."[1] But though the new law and the multibillion-dollar Albany Mall were probably the choicest items in the legacy of the perennial candidate and ex-governor Nelson Rockefeller, it doesn't seem as if the law had more than a marginal impact on the drug scene.[2] Some dealers who specialized in marijuana and occasionally sold a little coke decided that since the narcs weren't really bothering the grass sellers but were hot to get anyone connected with cocaine, it was good business to stick to their specialty and leave cocaine to those who were willing to risk big jail sentences. This initial small-scale defection didn't much affect matters, except to inconvenience those customers who had to look for a new coke dealer. The regular coke dealers certainly didn't close up shop, they simply used the new law as an excuse to boost prices and cut quality. And before many months had passed they realized the new law had, if anything, made them safer from arrest and conviction than they had been under the previous less stringent one. Far fewer arrests were being made[3] and, if previous history was any indication, juries would be reluctant to convict a man for selling say a half-ounce of coke when it meant sending him to prison for life.[4]

No, what really changed the New York situation is best explained by Gresham's Law—bad money drives out good. In this case, bad cocaine drove out good cocaine or, more to the point, the bad dealers drove out the good dealers. To see how this happened requires an understanding of the situation prior to the runaway inflation, when three distinct cocaine markets operated in New York.

The oldest continuing floating crap game of them all is in Harlem. When cocaine seemed to have virtually disappeared from the white areas of the city between 1930 and 1950, it was still around in Harlem. But, as I have previously mentioned, the Harlem market provided neither quality cocaine nor good prices. While a white middle-class cocaine buyer could buy a pure gram for $50 in 1970, his Harlem counterpart had to pay $50 for a 25 per cent gram. The Harlem dealers weren't noticeably greedier than their midtown colleagues, but they didn't have lines to the primary cocaine sources in South America. They had to go to the organized crime drug people for their supplies, and you don't get a square deal from the Mafia. They ripped the black dealers off just as they rip off everyone they do business with. (The situation has changed now that blacks have become a potent force in organized crime. Big black dealers have pure coke; which doesn't mean their customers get it, but that's another story.) At any rate, buying coke in Harlem was a fool's game unless that was where you *had* to buy it.

The white middle-class coke scene was quite a different matter. Up through 1971 good cocaine was readily available at reasonable prices, reasonable at least when you consider the prices for bad coke uptown. And the white buyer who had been smoking grass for a while and decided he'd like to try coke didn't have to hunt up a new dealer. His old, established neighborhood grass dealer was the man. And just as he usually could be counted on to have good grass, good acid, good whatever—he could usually

145

be counted on to have good coke, chiefly because his supplier was the same guy who delivered the rest of his goods. (The one thing you could almost never get from a typical grass dealer was heroin. They didn't use it and wouldn't sell it. Nor would their supplier.) But how did a low-level dealer's connection get cocaine in the first place?

To begin with, most of the grass sold in America comes from Mexico, and it enters the country in very large shipments—by the ton. In the early 1960s when grass was still a novelty to most people, the shipments were on a much smaller scale. As the demand for grass grew, the importer's operations grew, and as they grew they became more organized and more profitable. By 1966 or so there were several very large grass operations, most of them based in California. The people running them naturally developed close working relationships with the Mexican growers, and when some of the importer's customers began asking for cocaine, the importers went to their Mexican business friends. Can you get me coke? Of course they could. If they didn't sell it themselves, they knew someone who did. The Mexicans, after all, had long had connections with the South American cocaine market. (The first time I ever saw cocaine was in 1955 when the son of a rich Mexico City businessman passed it out, along with the joints, at a party. It was his first trip to the United States and he was surprised, almost unbelieving, that none of us had ever seen cocaine before. He said his father and his father's friends used it, but got quite upset when they suspected their sons of taking an occasional taste.) Anyway, the big grass importers added coke to their line of goods. About this same time they began bringing in the odd lot of Colombian grass, a premium product in the world of marijuana. At first they were getting it from their Mexican associates, but they soon developed sources in Colombia. Once this happened they were just a step away from the mother lode of Bolivian and Peruvian coke, and sitting in the middle of the Colombian market. They no longer had to go

146

through Mexican middlemen, they had direct access to primary cocaine sources, and some of them began to specialize in cocaine. It was a lot less hassle to bring in 50 kilos of coke than several tons of grass, and the profits were delicious. (In 1969 a kilo of pure Bolivian flake cost $1,500 at most in South America and could be sold for $12,500 in San Francisco.)

As cocaine grew more popular more people got into the importing act. Small dealers began making the trip to La Paz and bringing back a kilo or two to sell in retail quantities, thus eliminating the wholesaler. There were many such dealers in 1970 and 1971, and many more who bought small quantities from them, half-ounces and ounces. For a number of reasons—which we will go into in due course—their customers usually got a fair deal from them. The story of one now retired dealer of this type, a story I am reasonably certain is true, provides some insight into these operations and also illustrates how they came to an end.

This twenty-eight-year-old college graduate had been dealing grass, coke, and an assortment of psychedelics for several years and on a full-time basis between 1969 and 1972. At the end of 1971 he decided to give up dealing and go back to graduate school. But though he had lived well and traveled widely, had a nice apartment and a new car, he didn't have much money saved. About $6,000, nowhere near enough to get him through the three years of school he planned. So his supplier, an old friend, generously set him up with his Bolivian source. Carl invested in a round-trip ticket to La Paz and returned three weeks later with two $2,000 kilos of 91.2 per cent pure flake cocaine. He put aside 10 ounces, 20 grams for his personal use, presented the same quantity to the friend who made the connection for him, and set about selling the 60 remaining ounces—which he did in seven months, as follows:

Twenty one-ounce sales @ $800		$16,000
Eight ½-ounces @ $450		3,600
Fifty-six ¼-ounces @ $275		15,400
Six hundred and sixteen grams @ $50		30,800
		$65,800

After he finished this operation, Carl closed up shop and went back to school. But there is a lot more to his story than this bare outline, and here it is in his own words:

"It happened near the end, in July I think. I'd invested all my capital and taken the risk of bringing those kees in so that I could get out of this scene and finish my education in comfort. But you know how it is. Things go easy and you figure, I'll cut it down but no need to cut it *out*. Just do enough to pay expenses and when I'm finished school here's this nice bundle waiting for me. Invest it and watch it grow. So that's where my head was in July. There was only about five plus ounces left, most of it my personal stash. Well I'd been *hearing* things were getting heavy . . . I mean a couple of guys told stories about going to pick up a quarter-pound and having to sit at a table with a .45 automatic between them and the coke. And then there were some stories about guys coming in to make a pound buy, and ripping off the pound at the point of a gun. But I figured . . . Christ, they've got to be the worst kind of amateurs. I mean I would *never* buy from anyone I hadn't known a long, long time. The same goes for selling. I just do not sell to strangers. Period. I mean I took seven months to move those two kees. I just refused to take on a new customer. Not even when my best customers vouched totally for someone. They'd have to cop for them and that was that. No new faces. . . .

"So there I was sitting pretty in July. I'd made my rules and I stuck to them. I was invulnerable,

148

right? Wrong. One night I'm expecting a customer, and right on time the buzzer sings the right signal and I let him in. But it's not him, it's these two Latin dudes. . . . They walk right past me, sit down and say, 'We hear you have the very best cocaine.' I start saying, 'You've made a mistake,' and they smile and show me these big fucking guns. So I sit down. Then they break out some coke and very politely ask me to taste it. I'm not following the script at all but I take a taste. It's good rock coke with just a mild hit on it and I say something like very nice or whatever. Yes, they say, but *you* have the very *best*. We'd like to see it, all of it.

"Just about then the wild idea strikes me that these dudes are narcs, playing games. I say something about a warrant and they start giggling. . . . Which really gets to me. I start thinking of the old Richard Widmark movie I'd seen a couple of nights before. . . . The one dude giggles so hard he has to wipe his eyes. When he finishes he fondles his gun and says whoever gave me this shouldn't worry you, what should worry you is that I have it. I saw his point and took them to the stash. Like I said there was just a little more than five ounces left so I wasn't too concerned about the coke but naturally my *book* was there too [his record book, listing buys and sales, and telephone numbers of customers and connections]. When we get back inside the apartment the dude who did all the talking gives it to me straight. And I tell you it blew my mind. He says I can keep the coke, his people aren't *thieves*. Some people are but not his people. He only wants the book. We are businessmen, he says, who need to expand the retail side of our business. Then he says that my chances for a long and happy life would be greatly improved if I retired from the coke business. I agreed right away, and I wasn't bullshitting, and he knew I wasn't. I mean I was *scared,* man.

"And *then,* get this, he says, Ahh, I had forgotten, I need some of your excellent cocaine, how

149

much do you have for sale? For sale! and he's carrying a gun, he's ripped off my book, put me out of business and. . . . Well, I get a hold of myself and play it straight. I tell him I have very little for sale, five ounces are my personal stash. Weigh it, he says. I do and it comes to five ounces and six grams. Ahh, he says, almost a quarter. And how much is a quarter? $275 I say. Then $240 should be O.K. for six grams. Sure, that's fine, I say. Then he counts out some money and I give him the six grams. I put the money in my pocket, and he says you didn't count it! No, I say, under the circumstances it doesn't seem necessary. No, he says, our business is cocaine and we have just made a transaction—you should count the money. So I count it and it's only $180. He gives a big laugh and shakes his finger at me. Then he says a "friend" will deliver the balance in a few minutes, a "friend" named Roger. Roger is the guy I was expecting.

"Well, they leave and soon as they're out the door and down the stairs I phone up my supplier, the lovely dude who put me on to his connection in Bolivia, and tell him what went down. The only thing that surprises him is all the courtly cavalier business and the fact that they got to me who, after all, am a small-time dealer any way you look at it. He tells me that on his level this kind of thing has been going on for a while, though he never heard of anything so *polite* before. Which is why *he* got out of the business. They never got to him but he couldn't see staying in a scene so serious that dudes carried guns. And *used* them. He tells me that I must be under a very auspicious aspect, because every guy that's been hit that he's heard about has been totally ripped off, and a few of them have been killed. What *kind* of dudes were they, what nationality? he asks. Latin guys, I say. Yeah, he says, all this crap is being done by Cubans.

"Well, I sat for a couple of minutes trying to put it together. I mean I could understand them wanting the book, I had a select list of customers. But

150

leaving five ounces of the best coke and *buying* six grams just didn't make any sense. It still doesn't. The only thing I can think of is that the talkative dude had a little authority and was doing some kind of trip on the other guy. Like showing him you could be a coke dealer *and* a gentleman. Or maybe he wanted to get the word around that all you had to do was *cooperate* and nothing too serious would happen. I don't know, it was weird. Anyway, Roger showed up pretty soon and he was still shaking. What happened was that he was at a party and this Latin guy is passing coke around. Roger is an asshole at heart, so he breaks out *his* coke to one-up the guy. My coke is better than your coke.

"After a while the Latin dude gets him over in a corner and says, hey man, where can I get some of *that*? Roger tells him he can't 'cause the dealer won't sell to anyone he doesn't know personally. So the Latin dude says, look man, I've got a boss who is a connoisseur, you dig? He regards this coke of mine, the best rock coke, as shit. Can you imagine that? I would like to get him a taste of such fine cocaine. He would look on me with more regard. If you buy me a gram, I'll give you a gram of my coke for your trouble. Roger, being a greedy pig and no connoisseur, goes for it and tells the guy he can do it this very night, he's got an appointment at 10:30. So the guy gives him $60 and says he'll meet him back at the party at midnight. It's only 9:45 or so and Roger circulates a bit more.

"Meanwhile the Latin dude has obviously made a phone call because when Roger leaves about 10:15, the guy just happens to leave with him, saying he's got some business uptown and he'll meet him later as arranged. Roger is so dumb that this doesn't strike him as anything unusual. . . . Well I guess it wouldn't, except the guy had fronted Roger $60 to buy him a gram, and he'd never seen Roger before in his life. And that isn't kosher, but then Roger isn't exactly bright. Anyway, when they get downstairs the dude grabs Roger by the arm, puts a gun on him, and walks him to a car where there's two other Latin dudes, the ones that visited me. You know the rest."[5]

Minus the unlikely we-are-honorable-men-of-business motif, such episodes were not uncommon in New York between 1971 and 1973. The modus operandi varied considerably but the end result was the same, the decimation of a whole class of dealers. The Cubans who put Carl and his kind out of the coke business had been selling coke long before the white grass and coke dealers had ever smoked a joint. In pre-Castro times they operated out of Havana. After the revolution, those who had not been long gone figured prominently on the lists of undesirables Castro was happy to see come to America. He didn't want them, but being "anti-Communist," they were welcomed here. If they didn't like Castro, they must be good guys. They obviously weren't good guys, but they had very good connections in Bolivia and Peru, and when they got to Miami, they did what they had always done— sell coke. And made Miami the prime port of entry for South American cocaine.[6]

The biggest retail market for anything in the way of consumer goods is New York, and so the Cubans brought their goods north. At first their operations were confined to fellow expatriates and Puerto Ricans, but when cocaine entered the boom years of the early 1970s they naturally wanted to get a piece of the new action. Being organized criminals, they went about this in the traditional way—by muscling in on existing situations. Law enforcement people say there has been a war between the Cubans, blacks, and the Mafia with the Mafia coming out on the short end in the cocaine trade. The blacks service the Harlem and other black markets as they did before, but now they truly control it, having acquired primary cocaine sources in South America; the Cubans emerged as the most important group in the trade, controlling most of the East Coast and wholesaling to connections in Chicago, St. Louis, Kansas City, and Topeka.[7] Having no firsthand information on this subject, I can't vouch for its truth, but I do know that it was the Cubans who drove out most of the white middle-class cocaine dealers in New York.

The forcible acquisition of customer lists may strike the reader as a rather mild form of warfare for criminal gangs to indulge in. Keep in mind, however, that whatever else it is, selling cocaine is a business—and remember the great and devious lengths to which big corporations have gone to acquire a rival's mailing list. The Cubans were motivated by the same reason that led ITT to acquire the Hartford Insurance Company: increased profits. They had access to more cocaine than they could move in the Latin community, and the biggest and choicest market was composed of affluent whites, a market largely serviced by a network of independent white dealers. The Cubans wanted this market, and it was a safe and easy one to move in on. The hippy and Madison Avenue hippy dealers they decided to replace were not dangerous adversaries who would shoot it out with them as the blacks and the Mafia had been doing. These easy pigeons were criminals only in that they dealt in illegal products. They weren't the kind of people who, when forced out of one criminal endeavor, would simply turn to another like car theft, bank robbery, and the like. If they all weren't true members of the counter-culture, they all believed they were. And hardly any of them could seriously imagine doing business at the point of a gun, or have the desire to do it.

The drastic reduction in the availability of high quality cocaine in the East resulted directly from this take-over by organized crime. Not that the replaced dealers had sold nothing but good cocaine, that they rarely moved a bad product. Many prided themselves on providing quality but many took their customers for as much as they could get away with. Still, high-quality cocaine was available in quantities as small as a gram until the Cubans controlled the affluent white market. Both the Cubans and those they pushed out sold cocaine to make money, but as maximizers of profit the old-line dealers operated under a built-in disadvantage. For however greedy they may have been, they still regarded themselves as members in good standing of the antiestablishment drug culture, and ripping off fellow members to make as much money as possible did not fit this image. Most of them were not above selling the unknowing 40- to 50-per cent cocaine laced with a little speed as 80- to 90-per cent pure cocaine, but few of them could bring themselves to do this with 20- to 25-per cent cocaine. They could rationalize the first situation, but the second was too blatantly sour to indulge in and still retain one's self-image. The Cubans suffered from no such illusions. They didn't see themselves as serving a community to which they belonged and to whose values they must at least render lip-service. Their values were purely those of the marketplace—to provide only as much quality as was consistent with maximizing profits and staying in business.

Since, unlike heroin, cocaine is not a drug the user *must* have, one might think that once good quality had virtually disappeared, the customers would refuse to make do with inferior goods. But this is not the way the world works. Some users refused to buy bad cocaine just as some food shoppers refuse to buy bad produce in their local supermarket, but most coke users resigned themselves to the situation. There wasn't much else they could do unless they were willing to give up cocaine altogether. It is difficult to organize boycotts against legal products, it is impossible to do so against illegal ones. Outraged cocaine buyers can hardly set up a picket line around a dealer's establishment.

The present situation, then, is that where the cocaine trade is largely in the hands of organized crime, the product is inferior and the prices very high. According to both law enforcement officials and coke buyers, this is the prevailing state of affairs in the East and Midwest. At the moment the West Coast situation is quite different. For one reason or another, organized crime has never been firmly entrenched in the drug markets of Los Angeles and San Francisco, and the trade there is still largely in the hands of the old independent dealers. Good quality cocaine is not a rarity, and the prices are significantly lower than in the East. Ounces of pure cocaine are available in Los Angeles at $1,500, and for somewhat less in San Francisco. Recently, a new influx of moneyed Hollywood people into the market has apparently driven up prices in Los Angeles.

Whatever the quality, the prices are by any standard outrageous. Legal pharmaceutical cocaine—1,057 kilos of which were manufactured in the U.S. in 1969—sells for about $20 an ounce.[8] Similarly legal heroin in England costs less than 10 cents a grain, whereas illicit heroin in New York runs about $14 per grain when bought in standard $5 bags.[9] The reason for this vast price differential is, of course, that the black marketeer can charge whatever the traffic will bear. That heroin addicts will pay such prices is understandable, they are addicted, and their choices severely limited; but cocaine users are not addicted, they do not need cocaine to stave off withdrawal pains, and yet they pay fantastic prices. Some very tiny percentage of them may be so psychologically dependent on the drug that they are willing to pay any price, but these are exceptional cases and certainly too few in number to keep prices at such a high level. The great majority of regular users, moreover, are moderates who regard cocaine as a special treat to be used only a few times a month. All in all, then, the prices paid for cocaine don't seem to make much sense.

Most drug "authorities" argue that the psychic dependence induced by cocaine is so great that the depression suffered in the wake of abrupt secession is severe enough to class cocaine withdrawal with that from heroin and alcohol. And thus, according to them, the high prices do make sense. This is not sense but nonsense. To begin with, the best evidence available—the reports of users and studies made of large cocaine-

155

using populations—makes it clear that dependence on cocaine is an unusual phenomenon.[10] And secondly, even if one assumed that most cocaine users were heavily dependent on the drug, this false assumption would not explain the high cost of cocaine. For not even the most ardent critics of cocaine will argue that cocaine dependence is any more powerful than that produced by the amphetamines. Indeed, few would argue that it is as great. Yet the amphetamines, at the very height of their popularity, were only a tiny fraction of the cost of cocaine.

Scarcity is another argument put forth to account for the price of cocaine. But since even the narcs agree that there is more cocaine around than ever before, this is hardly a persuasive argument. Moreover, there is no shortage of coca leaves in the world and, given the current size of the cocaine market, the profits made in it, and the ever growing demand for cocaine, there is certainly no lack of incentive for setting up additional refineries if they are needed.

The most persuasive though far from satisfactory explanation of the high cost of cocaine centers around its snob appeal. It is and has been, since the upper classes took it over from the working classes, the most "in" drug available and the drug which conferred most status on the user. To pay good money for a subtle, short-lived experience is the mark of one who appreciates the finer things in life. To pay a lot of money for an experience the typical novice does not even perceive is the mark of a connoisseur. Once cocaine acquired this reputation, the steep rise in price was probably inevitable: tradesmen are always quick to understand what can be charged for a product which sets the buyer apart from the multitudes. (If you doubt this, consult a Neiman-Marcus Christmas catalog.) And once the price of cocaine was pegged high enough to serve this purpose, other snob appeal factors entered to boost it further. For being able to afford cocaine not only sets one apart from the masses, it marks the user as a success in his chosen field whether he be a garment salesman, musician, or dealer. And to be able to provide your guests with cocaine is both a gesture of the utmost chic and a way of displaying a standard of living far beyond the ordinary. The ability to provide such satisfactions, however artificial they may be, always commands a high price.

Some appreciation of just how expensive cocaine really is can be gained by comparing it with heroin. In New York at this writing, good cocaine is selling for $1,800 to $2,000 an ounce, good heroin for $1,000 to $1,200. But an ounce-against-ounce comparison is very misleading. On the value scale which truly counts —the length of time a user can stay high on his drug of choice—cocaine is considerably more than half again as expensive as heroin. For unlike heroin (four to six hours), LSD (eight to ten hours), or the amphetamines (four to six hours), cocaine's most notable effects last only about thirty minutes. The heroin user who can afford ounce quantities pays approximately $2.75 per grain and one-third of a grain will keep him high four to six hours. The cocaine user who can buy ounces pays approximately $4.00 per grain, and one-third of a grain will keep him high for thirty minutes. On a cost-effectiveness scale, therefore, cocaine is at least twelve times as expensive as heroin. On the more common street level of buying, where the heroin and cocaine has been heavily adulterated, the consumer pays a much higher price but the cost-effectiveness ratio remains about the same.

If the unreasonable price structure, the increasing incidence of violence, and the severe penalties imposed for possessing cocaine, are not enough to discourage the prospective cocaine buyer, the thoroughly dishonest practices of the marketplace should at least lead him into despair and great caution. Caveat emptor applies with a vengeance.

Good quality cocaine is not as rare elsewhere as it is in New York, but it undoubtedly will be in the near future. Dealers as a class simply cannot resist selling the affluent novices who have come into the market bad merchandise at high prices. And once a merchant discovers he can make money selling inferior goods, it is hard for him to return to the old ways.

The innocent might think that given the price of cocaine they would at least get what they paid for, but illicit drugs are not covered by Fair Trade rules or the Pure Food and Drug Act. Even so seemingly straightforward a matter as the weight of the purchase is no straightforward matter at all. When the purchase is an ounce or more, the material usually weighs what it is supposed to weigh. The dealer expects such a buyer to be careful and knowledgeable enough to have his own accurate scales. Thus an ounce will almost always be a full 28 grams. Gram buyers, on the other hand, can expect to be shortchanged. Few grams ever weigh a gram. And when you get down to a "spoon," the most common quantity sold, you enter a thoroughly nebulous area. A spoon may range anywhere from one-sixteenth to one-half of a teaspoon, though one-quarter teaspoon (slightly more than one-half gram) is the supposed standard.

The problems of measurement, however, are but a minor irritant. What really matters is how much cocaine the sample contains—and here all retail buyers face much the same problems. The ounce buyer has a far greater chance of obtaining relatively pure coke for his money than the spoon buyer who has virtually no chance at all, but he has no *assurance* that what he receives is pure cocaine. The questions for all buyers, therefore, are how pure is this cocaine, and what has it been cut with? Lacking a chemical laboratory, these are not easy questions to answer. Essentially, the average buyer must rely on four simple empirical tests, none of which alone is conclusive and which even in concert are not foolproof.

The Appearance of Cocaine

(In what follows "refined cocaine" refers to illicit cocaine, which when "pure" runs from 85 to 92 per cent cocaine; "pharmaceutical cocaine" is legal cocaine

158

refined to the point where it is 100 per cent cocaine. These and other technical questions are discussed in Appendix IV.)

Refined cocaine comes in two forms, rock and flake, the latter being a purer cocaine obtained by subjecting the rock form to an additional refining step. (Pharmaceutical cocaine is always flake.) Flake cocaine roughly resembles tiny snow crystals, if you can imagine hard snow. Rocks are usually the size of small irregular pebbles but may be as big as golf balls—though no retail buyer is likely to see one of this size. In both forms, uncut cocaine has a shiny, almost transparent look. And when crushed into powder—the form of cocaine most small buyers see insofar as powder facilitates the cutting process—uncut cocaine still retains a dull sparkle.

As proof of purity, a dealer will often point to the rocks in the sample being shown. If he takes a razor blade and slices the rock open, revealing crystalline layers the rock is a pure rock. If he does not, the matter is in doubt. It is not unusual for cut cocaine to be reconstituted into rocks.

Most of the commonly used cuts dull the sparkle of pure cocaine, and all of them change its appearance to some degree. Boric acid and methedrine crystals (a meta-amphetamine) most resemble cocaine and are the hardest to detect by visual examination. The sugar cuts, such as dextrose and lactose, dull cocaine's sparkle more than most cuts. Salts, such as quinine and Epsom, have a crystalline structure, but the crystals are less shiny than those of cocaine. Procaine, lidocaine, tetracaine, and benzocaine—all of which are local anesthetics used as cocaine substitutes but lack its stimulant properties—are crystalline in structure and shiny but, not being easy to get, are not very popular cuts. When they are used they are difficult to detect by eye. It is a common belief among cocaine users that the cutting agents reduce the longevity of the drug. This is not true. Cocaine is a stable alkaloid, retains its full potency for years, and the cuts do not affect its longevity.

The Taste of Cocaine

(In coke parlance, taste means sample; but here the word is used literally.)

As the various cuts alter the appearance of cocaine, so do they change its taste and its effect on the tongue. Pure cocaine has a bitter medicinal flavor, less astringent, for example, than alum but more so than lemon. The sugar cuts sweeten the taste, but lactose less than dextrose. (Dextrose on the other hand dulls the sparkle less than lactose.) The salt cuts are decidedly more bitter than cocaine. The synthetic local anesthetics are about equally bitter, but they numb the tongue more quickly and the numbness lasts longer. Neither the sugar nor salt cuts have any numbing effect and thus, if they are present, will reduce this effect of cocaine in relation to the amount of the cut.

Clearly both visual observation and tasting are at best crude instruments for determining the purity of cocaine—requiring as they do delicate distinctions without benefit of a standard—crude, however, only in the sense of not being objectively verifiable. They are analogous, in fact, to wine-tasting, an art dependent on the experience and sensitivity of the individual taster. No connoisseur of wine will mistake Ripple for Lafitte-Rothschild '69, and no connoisseur of cocaine will mistake 50 per cent coke for 92 per cent coke; but both are subject to error when finer distinctions must be made. Subjecting a sample of cocaine to the burn test is another step in reducing error.

The Burning of Cocaine

This is done by placing a small, measured amount of cocaine on a piece of aluminum foil and holding it over a low flame. Pure pharmaceutical cocaine burns

160

clear, leaving no residue. Refined cocaine leaves a reddish brown stain on the foil and a small amount of residue. This residue constitutes various impurities (chiefly other alkaloids) which remain in refined cocaine but which have been eliminated from pharmaceutical cocaine. In either case sugar cuts will darken the burn and the larger the cut the darker the burn. The stain remaining from pharmaceutical cocaine cut with sugar is dark brown or black, that from refined cocaine black. Salt cuts do not burn and remain as residue. Thus if half the burn sample remains as residue you can be sure you have no more than 50 per cent cocaine. Unfortunately, and quite apart from the cuts that leave no residue but change the color of the burn, there are several cuts which burn clear and leave no residue. Methadrine crystal, the synthetic local anesthetics, quinine, and menita all behave this way. Unlike cocaine, however, procaine and the other synthetics bubble noticeably before disappearing. And methadrine crystal sizzles and pops.

Though the burn test is more objective than visual observation and tasting, it too is a good deal less than foolproof. There are more sophisticated tests for which laboratory equipment is not required—methanol, cobalt, and volume differentiation—and these are given in Appendix VII. But short of these or chemical analysis, the surest way to ascertain the potency of a sample of cocaine is to use it. That is, to snort it.

Snorting Cocaine

While the surest method, this is also the most subjective. No one reacts precisely the same way to anything, and the varieties of response to cocaine vary widely among individuals. Moreover, there are certain gross reactions detectable by the attentive novice, and there are subtle ones no novice is likely to detect.

If a snort burns the nasal passage and brings tears

to the eyes, the chances are that a methadrine cut has been used. Many novices, however, react this way the first time they snort pure cocaine. If shortly after a couple of moderate snorts, one detects a notable postnasal drip, the chances are that one of the many sugar or salt cuts is present. And if an evening of moderate cocaine indulgence results in pronounced diarrhea, it's a good bet that the cocaine was cut with Epsom salts or menita, both of which are laxatives.

These reactions could be noted by a novice, as could the excessive sweating and hyperactivity produced by methadrine or quinine cuts. At this point, however, the need of past experience becomes stronger. For how can someone unfamiliar with cocaine tell if the increased energy he feels is the result of cocaine or speed? If he is familiar with speed, he might make a very educated guess; if not, he can't tell. But if a couple of hours after two moderate snorts, you are still being far more active than usual, it is very likely that the cocaine was generously cut with speed. And if the "freeze"—that numbness which follows a snort of cocaine and which is particularly noticeable in the nose and the upper front gums—is felt distinctly more than one-half an hour after a snort, you can be sure that one of the local anesthetics was used as a cut.

But the most important consideration in determining the quality of cocaine by snorting is the quality of the resulting high. It is also the one most subject to error and difference of opinion. There are three distinct components to a cocaine high: increased energy, clarity of mind, and euphoria. The precise blend of these qualities and the extent to which they are experienced both singly and collectively are controlled by both the purity of the cocaine and the character of the individual. But even the same person will not react to the same cocaine the same way on every occasion. Our moods and metabolism fluctuate continually, and both affect the quality of the high we experience. Consequently, to reliably ascertain the purity of cocaine by snorting requires a developed sensitivity, the cataloguing of past experience, and a close attention to present details. In short one must be a connoisseur.

Indeed it should be apparent by now that these simple tests provide the average user with only gross indications. The only people capable of employing them with a high degree of accuracy are experienced cocaine users who have paid close attention to their experience. But gross indications are better than none. For without these tests, or those listed in the appendix, the buyer must rely on the dealer. Some dealers are reliable, most are not.

8

The Effects of Cocaine

Considering the extravagantly high price of cocaine, the slim chances of procuring anything resembling a quality product, the special attention given it by narcotics officers, and the fact that its devotees are not, like heroin users, in bondage to their drug, it is obvious that unless cocaine afforded very marked pleasures its current popularity would be inexplicable. That cocaine does offer such pleasures is beyond dispute. Equally indisputable is the fact that a very small number of users experience seriously unpleasant reactions and a goodly number of regular users experience mildly unpleasant reactions when they overindulge. To understand these differing reactions requires some understanding of cocaine's action on humans.

The effects of cocaine, or any other drug, can be roughly divided into three categories: physiological, how it acts on the various systems of the body; psychoactive, how it affects feelings, mood, and behavior; and, applicable to both, the reactions resulting from either an unusual sensitivity to the drug, from very high doses, or from chronic long-term use which may be classed under the rubric of adverse and/or toxic reactions. Since the most common adverse reactions are inextricably linked to how cocaine affects individual users, it makes more sense in my view to discuss them along with the positive psychoactive effects rather than under a separate heading. At the same time there are a few notable, if uncommon, toxic reactions which merit special attention: these will be discussed following the section on the psychoactive effects of cocaine.

Enough has already been said about the effects of cocaine to make it clear that the reports of users disagree violently with the pronouncements of certified drug authorities, few of whom have ever taken cocaine. The one area in which there is little disagreement is that of the physiological effects. This area, a technical one, may be of small interest to the average reader but since what *is* known is generally agreed on, it seems appropriate to give this information before getting into the more interesting and controversial area of cocaine's psychoactive effects.

Physiological Effects I

Described below are the gross bodily effects of cocaine. Those interested in the technical details relating to the distribution and fate of cocaine in the body, together with its effects on the sympathetic nervous system should consult "The Psychopharmacology of Cocaine" by James H. Woods and David A. Downs, in which the authors present a careful review of the relevant medical literature.[1]

Absorption: The most efficient way of introducing cocaine into the body is by intravenous injections. The highest blood levels of cocaine and the most noticeable behavioral effects are produced by this route.[2] (There are no research data on the relationship between blood levels and behavioral effects, however.)

165

But except among heroin and methadone users who also use cocaine, intravenous injection of cocaine is rare. The most inefficient route of administration is by mouth, cocaine being poorly absorbed into the bloodstream from the gastrointestinal tract.[3] Once a very common way of taking cocaine, it is now almost nonexistent. (Indian coca-chewers don't really use this oral route. They chew and suck on a quid of leaves, so most of their cocaine intake is through the mucous membranes of the mouth and throat.) Subcutaneous and intramuscular injections are also inefficient routes of administration.[4] The most common method of taking cocaine, snorting it through the nasal passages, is also a very efficient route of administration, passing quickly through the mucous membranes of the nose and throat into the bloodstream.[5] (Smoking cocaine— putting cocaine on the end of a cigarette or sprinkling it throughout a joint—is a practice enjoying something of a vogue. There is no technical information respecting its efficiency. Anecdotal evidence, however, suggests that it is a relatively efficient route.)

Distribution: The way in which cocaine is distributed to the various tissues of the body following administration has not been studied in man. In dogs, the highest concentrations of cocaine are found in the spleen, kidney, and cerebral cortex; considerably smaller amounts are in the heart, skeletal muscles, liver, fat, pancreas, and blood plasma.[6]

Fate: The action of cocaine in the body is terminated by three mechanisms: metabolism, excretion via the urine, and distribution to inactive sites. Metabolism appears to be the major mechanism, but very little is known about cocaine metabolism and, consequently, little is known about distribution to inactive sites.[7]

Little more is known about the excretion of cocaine via the urine. Studies have reported anywhere from 1 to 21 per cent unchanged cocaine in urine samples,[8] a range so wide as to indicate a very complex situation. So little is known about this that interpretation of its significance is impossible.

Most of the cocaine in the body is detoxified by

the liver at a rate which has been estimated at one minimal lethal dose per hour.[9] Since most texts concur that the lethal dose is 1.2 grams, this is apparently the amount detoxified by the liver in an hour—but this is obviously only a rough estimate.

Tolerance and Physical Dependence: In what I would term "true addiction," exemplified by addiction of the opiate type, at least two conditions must be present: (1) tolerance, which is shown by a reduction of the effects of a given dose after repeated administration. Put another way, to achieve the same effects the user must escalate dosage; and (2) physical dependence, which is indicated by noticeable withdrawal symptoms following discontinuation of the drug.

Neither tolerance nor physical dependence occur with cocaine. The same dose will produce the same effects after repeated administration, and no noticeable withdrawal symptoms are evident when the drug is discontinued.[10]

Physiological Effects II

The most striking clinical action of cocaine is its ability to block nerve conduction when applied locally, i.e., its efficiency as a local anesthetic. Its most striking general effect is stimulation of the central nervous system.

Central Nervous System Effects: The first recognizable action is on the cerebral cortex and is manifested in humans by psychic stimulation and increased motor activity which remains well coordinated under low doses. As the dose is increased, the lower centers of the brain are stimulated, and this can cause tremors and convulsive movements. Large doses can cause depression of the CNS either as a result of cocaine-induced convulsions or as the immediate effect of high concentrations of cocaine reaching the brain.[11] Low and moderate doses increase the respiratory rate, with little effect on the depth of respiration. Large doses may result in rapid, shallow breathing, and even respiratory failure.[12] Very few such cases have ever been reported, and none in recent times.

(The pharmacological texts I have consulted repeatedly refer to "low," "moderate," and "large" doses without ever defining what is meant by these terms—a defect which indicates far less data than the authoritarian tone of their pronouncements would lead one to expect.[13] The term "low dose" apparently refers to the average doses taken by coca-chewing Indians, but since they, in fact, ingest several times as much cocaine as the text writers have long believed—an average of 6 grains per day rather than 0.6 grains—all the data supposedly gathered on low-dose effects are probably invalid. Coca chewing does in all likelihood result in a slower absorption rate of cocaine than does snorting, and hence there are undoubtedly significant differences between the effects of snorting and chewing like amounts—though not so great as the difference between snorting and swallowing cocaine, since much of the cocaine entering the bloodstream of coca chewers comes through the mucous membranes of the mouth and throat rather than from the gastrointestinal tract. However this may be, I *assume* that "moderate" refers to the typical 20- to 30-milligram dose snorted by the average user every 30 minutes to one hour, and that "large" refers to the 50- to 100-milligram doses injected every ten minutes or so by heavy intravenous users or to the single large (800-milligram)[14] doses sometimes given in medical contexts.)

Cardio-Vascular Effects: Cocaine directly affects the heart and blood vessels. Due to the vasoconstrictive action of the drug, blood pressure rises when cocaine is first introduced to the body and returns to normal as the effects wear off. Small doses slow the heart rate, moderate doses increase it. Large doses may result in cardiac failure due to a direct toxic reaction on the heart.[15] No such fatal reactions have been reported among recreational users.

Muscular Effects: There is certainly a subjective feeling that muscular strength is increased, but since Freud

168

demonstrated increased muscular strength way back in 1884,[16] to my knowledge no research has been conducted in this area.

Body Temperature: Body temperature rises. The contributing factors are thought to be vasoconstriction (which decreases heat loss), increased muscular activity, and possibly the effect of cocaine on the heart-regulating centers.[17]

Other Physiological Effects: At least three effects of cocaine are reported by almost all users which are of some interest. (1) When snorted, the vasoconstrictive properties of the drug cause a marked drying up of the mucous membranes. For those suffering from colds or sinusitis, this brings initial relief. Repeated doses, however, usually result in blocked nasal passages. (2) Cocaine is apparently a natural laxative and increased bowel movements are the rule. And (3) it also seems to stimulate the bladder and increased urination is common.

And, of course, cocaine numbs the nose, palate, and gums of all snorters as well as any other area to which it is applied.

Psychoactive Effects

Introduction: If there is little good data available on cocaine's physiological effects, there is a great deal available on its psychoactive effects. But there are almost no such data from controlled investigations. Freud made the first careful study of the psychoactive effects of cocaine by closely observing his own reactions, but most modern researchers reject such efforts as being too subject to the personal bias of the investigator. For the same reasons, they put little faith in the reports of observers. And insofar as the reports from both users and observers range from the ecstatic to the horrified, their skepticism appears warranted. Or would be warranted—though mistaken as I shall later argue—if they treated all subjective reports in the same way. But this is not the case. Where illicit drugs are concerned, the prevailing practice is to accept the most adverse reports and then to elevate them to generalities applicable to all users. This is not only unscientific, it is dishonest.

As for the larger question of what is the best information available for evaluating the psychoactive effects of drugs, the answer surely is that the primary and most important source is the reports of users. Indeed who else *but* the user can tell us how a specific drug and dosage affects feelings and moods? For these effects *are* subjective and can be described only by the person experiencing them. And this brings to mind another difficulty inherent in a research philosophy which insists that subjective involvement destroys objectivity to the point where all results are, if not completely invalid, too suspect to be valuable: namely, the inability of drug-innocent researchers to properly assess the reports of users. The problem here is that such observers—a category to which almost all current pharmacological authorities belong—have no standard against which to measure these reports other than that provided by analogy, and analogy is frequently misleading, to say the least. For example, the term "hallucinogen" was applied to LSD by LSD-innocent researchers who, from the reports of users, were led to believe that the drug induced hallucinations. The users, however, didn't report they were having hallucinations, they reported visual and auditory imagery and tactile sensations which the researchers *interpreted* as hallucinations. When researchers began taking LSD themselves, they discovered the mistake. For what they heard, saw, and felt under the drug lacked a necessary condition of hallucinatory experience—the belief that what is being experienced *is* the structure of reality. They also learned that like themselves, the nonscientific users were perfectly aware they were not experiencing hallucinations.

There is more to be said on this question but before doing so, let us first consider the psychoactive effects of cocaine as reported by users and then as reported by the pharmacological researchers.

Effects Reported By Users (with a few nods to the researchers): Both researchers and users agree that cocaine produces euphoria, sexual stimulation, increased energy, and reduces fatigue and appetite. Users also insist that it increases mental lucidity and muscular strength, but most researchers believe that users simply "feel" this way rather than actually have these attributes. Those researchers who have used cocaine agree with the users.[18]

The speed with which these effects are experienced, and their duration, depends chiefly on the mode of administration. Intravenous injection produces the effects almost instantaneously, and they endure in a pronounced way for about ten minutes. Snorting cocaine delays the full effects for a couple of minutes but they last for about thirty minutes in most cases. If one pays close attention to the effects, however, they can be felt in diminished form some two hours after inhaling a dose of 20 to 30 milligrams.

In general, the larger the dose, the more pronounced the effects. But large chronic doses usually lead to adverse results: euphoria may turn into anxiety, paranoia, and hallucinations; sexual stimulation to impotency; lucidity to confusion; and the lessening of fatigue to insomnia.

It must be stressed that there is a great diversity of individual reactions to cocaine, a fact rarely noted by researchers. Freud observed that some people reacted as he did, others experienced no reaction at all to small doses, and still others exhibited reactions much more marked than his own.[19] In interviewing and observing some 81 users who had access to high-quality cocaine (ranging from 70 to 92 per cent pure), I found, as Freud did, a wide variety of reactions.[20] All reported experiencing the effects listed in the first paragraph, but there was much variation respecting the degree to which particular effects were considered important. Some stressed feeling happy, some the sexual aspects of the drug, others were most impressed by the increase in energy they felt, and so on. All agreed, as might be expected, that cocaine was a

171

"good" drug, and virtually all were certain it should be used in moderation. There was considerable difference on what constituted moderate use. Some felt that snorting up a gram during the course of an evening once every two weeks or so was being moderate; some that a quarter to a half gram per day over a period of a few days was the intelligent approach to cocaine; others that this daily dosage over a period of a few weeks was proper; and a few felt that several grams a day was not excessive. All agreed that periods of abstinence were required as soon as any adverse effects were noted.

There was closer agreement on the nature of the adverse effects than on the positive effects. With the exception of one person who was apparently allergic to cocaine, and who experienced seriously depressed respiratory functions after snorting approximately one-tenth of a gram over a period of two hours, no moderate users—those who used one-quarter to one-half gram per day a few days at a time, or those who used upwards of a gram in an evening every two weeks or so—in a sample of 60 reported any adverse effects other than on those occasions when they used considerably more cocaine than usual. On such occasions, about three-quarters of the sample experienced feelings of lassitude the next day very like those felt during a mild alcoholic hangover.

Fourteen of 17 users who took cocaine in amounts of one-quarter to one-half gram per day on a regular, prolonged basis reported the following adverse effects appearing anywhere from two to five weeks after initiating use: mild insomnia; occasional impotency (But men are reluctant to admit impotency and, according to several of their lovers, this impotency was a good deal more than occasional); and the definite feeling that their personalities had been modified to the extent that they reacted more sharply to criticism, felt more impatient when faced with minor problems, and in general felt slightly on edge. These symptoms disappeared when they stopped using cocaine. And all but one said they had to experience these adverse effects at least twice before they were able to fully appreciate the importance of the warning signs and stick to their resolution to stop using cocaine for a week or two. Three of the moderate chronic users said they never experienced any adverse effects and only stopped using when their supply ran out.

The four heavy chronic users—from two to four grams a day—reported occasional adverse effects similar to those experienced by the moderates but in exaggerated form. And three of them reported feeling mildly paranoid after a couple of weeks of heavy use.

No one reported experiencing depression or marked craving for cocaine when their supply ran out. If they couldn't find any or couldn't afford to buy any, they simply did without. And no one felt they were dependent on cocaine. Apart from the comparison to heroin, and the quantities used, the following remarks might have been made by any of the users:

"I'm into coke all right. Anywhere from two to three grams a day, day in and day out except when my nose needs a rest. I'm careful about that. But I've never seen myself as *dependent* on it. I mean good coke isn't always around and I just won't use shit you see . . . so lots of times I have to go without it for weeks at a time. When my coke is gone and I can't get anything good, I just wait until it shows up. Sure I ask around, but I don't go scurrying all over town hunting for it. I mean I've never felt as if I *had* to have it. I like it, I like it a lot, but that's it believe me. Now smack, that's a different story. I once got into smack for a few months. I had what you'd call a very mild habit, about a couple of bags a day. But I felt I just had to have it no matter what. I was going to school at the time and didn't have much money so sometimes I'd steal money from my mother. I mean really *low* shit. I just can't imagine stealing money to buy cocaine. You really have to need something to steal for it; and cocaine just isn't that way."[21]

One other aspect of cocaine use as reported by these users is significant. Most say that when they first started they kept using more and more cocaine. That is, they escalated their dosages. In a short time, however, they realized they weren't feeling better and better, rather they were experiencing more and more adverse effects. Consequently, they cut down. They wanted the pleasures of cocaine, not the pains. And this moderation of use occurs in the great majority of cases. People learn from experience.

All these users like the effects of cocaine enough to spend considerable sums to indulge themselves. Many people, however, try cocaine and are not sufficiently impressed to spend money on it. For example, several lovers or friends of the regular users I observed remarked that though they occasionally used cocaine "because it was around," they didn't like it so much that they would go out and spend money to have it.

Effects Reported By Pharmacological Researchers: The literature on cocaine presents a story very different from that just given. Some typical examples:

"Cocaine is at first used occasionally for the sense of exhilaration and well-being it gives, but soon the depression and insomnia following the stimulation lead to a craving and later actual dependence on the drug."
—*The Practitioner's Library of Medicine and Surgery,* 1933[22]

"The stimulation [of cocaine] is succeeded by depression, tremors, pallor, sunken and unsteady eyes."
—*Manual of Pharmacology,* 1942[23]

"The repeated use of cocaine may lead to addiction. . . . The addict suffers an intolerable craving for the drug . . . and there is mental deterioration, leading ultimately to a state of permanent moral degeneracy."
—*British Pharmaceutical Codex,* 1963[24]

"Drug dependence of the cocaine type is . . . a state arising from repeated administration of co-

174

caine . . . on a periodic or continuous basis. Its characteristics include:

1. an over powering desire or need to continue taking the drug and to obtain it by any means;

4. . . . withdrawal is attended by a psychic disturbance manifested by craving for the drug."
—WHO Description of Drug Dependence of the Cocaine Type, 1964

"Both addiction and tolerance can result from the continued use of cocaine."
—*The Pharmacological Basis of Therapeutics,* 4th Ed., 1970[25]

"Cocaine produces a state of psychological exultation in man that is extremely strong and which involves feelings of euphoria. . . . Psychological depression, however, follows this state in a rather short period of time (30 minutes)."
—National Clearing House For Drug Abuse Information, 1972[26]

Apart from their authoritarian tone and unjustifiable generality, the common thread running through these quotations is the belief that cocaine is an addictive drug, because (1) withdrawal precipitates a severe psychological depression which can be overcome only by more cocaine, and (2) the user develops a craving for the drug. The facts, as we have seen, are quite different. Users neither report such depression nor such cravings. Why then do the "authorities" keep insisting they do? The answer, so far as I can tell, is that instead of experimenting on themselves or consulting current users, they have relied upon a handful of extreme cases carried in the literature since the time of Freud.

What is wrong with this practice is not the authorities' reliance on anecdotal evidence—anecdotal evidence being the most relevant evidence available on the psychoactive effects of drugs—but their use of extreme cases as the norm. And not only extreme cases, but ones of such vintage that no disinterested observer can verify them. Given the fact that information is available from current users, I can account for this dubious practice only by assuming that such authors either believe that the repetition of error leads to truth, or that they are doing their best to justify the idea that cocaine is an especially dangerous drug.

In either case they have had to work hard to do this. When cocaine was considered an addictive drug like the opiates, it was easy to affirm its especially dangerous nature; but once it was firmly established that no tolerance to cocaine was built, that no withdrawal symptoms worthy of the name occurred, and that in short cocaine could not be considered an addictive drug in the accepted meaning of the term, this was no longer easy to do in a scientifically respectable way. The same problem arose with marijuana, LSD, etc. To take care of these embarrassing situations, the drug experts substituted the notion of *dependence* for that of *addiction*: drugs which induced psychological dependence were obviously dangerous drugs, prohibitions against which were justifiable.[27] Of course, there still remained the vexing problem of defining "dependence" or, rather, demonstrating that specific drugs produced psychological dependence. With cocaine they decided, on the basis of a very small number of extreme cases, that the depression which followed abstinence was so great that the user saw cocaine as the only possible source of relief and, thus, if he was not physically dependent on cocaine he most certainly was psychologically dependent. As one author put it in 1972, ". . . cocaine withdrawal is characterized by a profound psychological manifestation—*depression*—for which cocaine itself appears to the user to be the only remedy. . . . The compulsion to resume cocaine is very strong."[28]

But as we have seen, the heavy depression which almost all current authorities insist follows the discontinuation of use is *not* a condition which any significant number of cocaine users have experienced. None of the 81 users I interviewed and observed experienced

176

any recognizable discomfort when their cocaine ran out beyond that feeling we all have when something we like is no longer at hand or readily available. Indeed even the heavy users voluntarily stopped for periods of time to get their noses back in shape and to avoid or relieve certain adverse reactions which usually accompany prolonged use. As for there being a strong compulsion to resume use, this is, as a general statement, devoid of meaning. Some users exhibit such a compulsion but in no case in my experience did it stem from a need to relieve depression. Rather, since cocaine is their drug of choice, such persons procure it whenever they can, finances permitting. Most users (60 out of 81), however, use cocaine in a very different manner. They like it and they use it on "special" occasions—in much the same way as one who regularly drinks wine with his dinner will occasionally treat himself and his guests to a fine vintage Bordeaux.

The ignorance of the effects of cocaine manifested by almost all pharmacologists, physicians, and drug experts is not irreversible. All that is required is honest attention to the reports of those best situated to know the effects of cocaine—the users. Indeed, in the past year two nationally recognized authorities who previously held views indistinguishable from those I have been criticizing have dramatically altered their opinions after consulting a number of users. Edward Brecher, the author of the Consumers Union Report *Licit & Illicit Drugs,* has recently written that "the deep depression following cocaine use described in my book—a depression which compels the user to return to cocaine—is . . . rare or nonexistent among cocaine users today."[29] And Dr. Norman Zinberg of Harvard University wrote that he previously had accepted the conventional descriptions of the harmfulness of cocaine, but that when he "began to study cocaine seriously" he found the facts to be quite different; he was unable to locate a single cocaine psychosis, nor did he find "the serious, profound depression upon cessation of use that is the standard description in the literature."[30]

(Officialdom is at last getting around to studying

177

the effects of cocaine on humans. After this book was in galleys, I came across a January, 1974 advertisement from The National Institute of Drug Abuse soliciting contract bids on nine proposed studies relating to cocaine use. Here is one of them:

Facts and Myths About Human Cocaine Use/ Abuse. The National Institute on Drug Abuse is soliciting source information from qualified organizations having the capability and facilities to investigate facts and myths about cocaine use/abuse. More specifically, this would involve an intensive literature search of the professional and lay literature as well as street myths relating to the effects of cocaine use. Moreover this would entail discussion of rituals of use, sharing behaviors, monetary costs, achieved statuses, and the mood states displayed by users both before, during and after use. This project would require sophisticated and broad ranged literature searches.

To qualify, organizations must give adequate evidence of (1) knowledge and experience in the psychosocial aspects of drug use/abuse, (2) clear documentation of research expertise in similar types of projects, with examples of methodologies used, and (3) availability of data sources with a description of the kinds of data to be collected. Responses must refer to SS NIDA-74-15. (RO14)

After so long a period of neglect, the NIDA's new interest in cocaine is to be commended. Unfortunately, nothing in the above proposal nor in the other eight leads me to suppose that the investigations will be conducted in anything but the usual way—that is, by persons with all the proper academic and bureaucratic credentials, but with no first-hand knowledge of cocaine, the kind of knowledge required to accurately interpret their data.

A few months prior to the issuance of this NIDA advertisement I attempted to secure a fellowship from the Ford Foundation's Drug Abuse Council in order to, and I quote, "examine and document the strong possibility that the ignorance which prevails among medical and pharmacological researchers regarding important aspects of the effects of specific drugs on individuals arises chiefly from the attempt to understand and describe these effects by 'objective' methods, methods made necessary by the need of researchers to conform to legal strictures and by the extra-legal pressures exerted on them by the Bureau of Narcotics and Dangerous Drugs and its predecessors." In short, I was saying that the ignorance displayed by researchers resulted from their lack of personal experience with the drugs they studied. I did not get the fellowship.

One other commonly promoted belief which should be put to rest is the erroneous notion that "Cocaine has the same effects as the amphetamines. The major difference is that the effects of the amphetamines last several hours, while those of cocaine seem to last only minutes."[31] Now this is a perfect example of the inadequacy of trying to understand the effects of drugs by the exclusive application of pharmacology. Objectively, or pharmacologically, cocaine and the amphetamines are very similar. Their subjective effects are, however, quite different. And this is not simply a difference in *duration,* it is a difference in *kind*. Cocaine is a subtle drug when ingested in the usual manner, i.e., by snorting; so subtle that naive users frequently need to have its effects pointed out to them before they can recognize them. (The response produced by injection is not subtle, but even here there is a great difference between the effects experienced in shooting cocaine and those experienced in shooting speed.) The amphetamines on the other hand are anything but subtle, and only that small handful of persons who paradoxically experience calming effects from the amphetamines would have the least difficulty recognizing their impact. Indeed persons who have thought they were using cocaine but were in fact using cocaine heavily cut with speed—a common street product these days—often charge a dealer with cheating them after he has sold them high-quality cocaine.[32]

They didn't experience the "kick" they had become accustomed to and which they had identified as the kick of cocaine.

But if cocaine is not the addictive, dependence-producing, dangerous drug it has been made out to be, it nevertheless can create serious toxic or adverse reactions. Such reactions are not common but as Freud once remarked, there are always those who will abuse any substance with which they come in contact.[33] Many of these reactions have already been noted, but a fuller discussion seems appropriate.

Toxic and/or Adverse Reactions To Cocaine

Shortly following cocaine's introduction as a local anesthetic in 1884, it was noted that it produced dangerous toxic reactions in some patients. An 1891 study listed 13 deaths but whether these were truly the result of cocaine or were due to a combination of factors is open to question.[34] A 1924 study listed an additional 26 deaths.[35] Two routes of administration seemed especially dangerous; topical application to the tonsils and insertion into the urethra. Most of these deaths occurred in medical situations, very few have ever been recorded from the social use of cocaine, and recent medical literature contains no cases at all of deaths among illicit cocaine users.[36] The frequent small doses which are the norm for the social user are clearly much safer than the single large doses by which physicians killed a number of patients.[37]

The lethal dose is usually estimated to be 1.2 grams, and severe toxic reactions are said to be possible with doses as small as 20 milligrams (1/50 gram).[38] Severe reactions to very small doses *are* possible, but to my knowledge occur only in those rare cases where the user is allergic to cocaine, one of which I have previously mentioned. No social user attempts doses of 1.2 grams. A heavy intravenous user might consume ten grams in a day but does so in doses of 50 to 100 milligrams. The cardiac arrests and respiratory failures resulting from large doses of cocaine have all occurred, so far as the literature shows, in medical settings.[39]

But to an allergic person an overdose can result from a very small amount. Moreover, death from an overdose of cocaine "is almost always prompt, and the accompanying physical signs represent a mixture of CNS stimulation, respiratory depression [the initial signs of which are rapid, shallow breathing] and cardio-vascular collapse. Convulsions are a common initial sign . . . but fainting is the first indication of trouble in many patients. Usually the heart continues to beat after respiration has ceased, but the heart's stopping first is not uncommon."[40] The course of cocaine's lethal action is so rapid that when any of the above signs are noted, resuscitative measures must be instituted immediately. There are no specific antidotes for cocaine poisoning, but the recommended nonspecific treatment is given in Appendix VI.

Though no lethal reactions have been reported among illicit users in modern times, adverse reactions following overindulgence are fairly frequent. Such reactions not only depend on the amount of cocaine consumed but are, as with the pleasurable effects, dependent on the individual. Some persons can consume several grams a day and experience no notable ill effects, while others experience them when they exceed a quarter of a gram. The point is that each user has an individual limit which when exceeded can lead to a variety of unpleasant reactions. Anxiety, insomnia, undue aggressiveness, paranoia, and hallucinations have all been reported by users who overdo it. The first three symptoms are not uncommon, the latter two are decidedly rare: true paranoid reactions and hallucinations are almost never reported by modern users, but the literature contains examples of both. In the hallucination cases, tactile ones—the sensation of insects or tiny animals crawling on or under the skin—are more common than the visual variety—persons or objects appearing smaller than normal.[41]

There are several warning signs which indicate that

the individual's dose limit is being exceeded: cold perspiration, excessive sweating, pallor, feelings of anxiety, exhibitions of aggressive behavior, insomnia, impotency, and feelings of heaviness in the limbs. All users should heed these signs. They indicate that the body contains more cocaine than it can safely handle, and a continued indulgence in cocaine may lead to an overdose.

Since the vast majority of cocaine users snort the drug, a tender nose is probably the most common adverse physical reaction to cocaine. The nose is lined with delicate mucous membranes and small hair follicles. Cocaine can lodge in these follicles and cause irritation, sores, and bleeding—conditions which are usually the result of too much cocaine or carelessness. Ignoring the conditions and continuing to snort cocaine may lead to a perforated septum, a serious and unpleasant consequence. In addition, cocaine may lodge in the sinus cavities, causing congestion and headaches.

Wise users take measures to prevent nasal and sinus problems. They keep their cocaine finely grained by chopping it with a razor blade or grinding it with a mortar and pestle. The finer the grain the less chance it will lodge in the nose or sinuses. Cautious users snort a little water after taking cocaine to dislodge or dissolve any bits held by the hair follicles. And the most prudent users rinse their noses thoroughly with warm water after snorting. Most users have found that the occasional use of nose drops or sprays is beneficial.

It should by now be absolutely clear that one cannot talk of the effects of cocaine in a manner which implies that the descriptions are applicable to all users. Individual responses are simply too varied to allow this. Why then, to return to our old question, have pharmacologists and other medical researchers generally written as if what happens to a few individuals on cocaine (and other psychoactive drugs for that matter) holds true for all or most individuals? And in so doing promulgated a vast body of cocaine mythology? The reason, I have suggested, is that they have refused to give proper weight to the accounts of users. And they have refused to do so chiefly because they have insisted on applying a scientific model which views subjective experience with great suspicion. The trouble with this "objective" approach is, as Andrew Weil has said, that ". . . it is impossible to talk meaningfully about the effects of psychoactive drugs, except by reference to their effects on specific individuals on specific occasions."[42]

In other words, the scientific model used by pharmacologists is totally inappropriate for the task of describing the psychoactive effects of drugs. For science is essentially the effort to find general rules which can both account for known facts and make predictions on the basis of known facts. And this effort is far more successful in some areas than in others. The less a science must concern itself with idiosyncratic individuals, the more successful it is in performing its essential function. Physics, for example, has been highly successful in generating general laws capable of precise predictions, whereas psychology has been largely unsuccessful. The reason, of course, is that people behave in ways far more eccentric than do atoms. Yet the desire to reduce experience to generalizations that we can easily understand and apply is powerful and leads to much unnecessary error. In 1973 upwards of 160,000 Americans died through overdoses or allergic reactions to prescribed drugs.[43] This did not happen because doctors are totally ignorant of the effects of drugs, but because they applied what is *generally* known about specific drugs to individuals who did not fit the general rules.

Such errors are to some extent unavoidable but one way of reducing their number and of generating a better understanding of the effects of drugs in general, is for the pharmacologists—one of whose major functions is the description of drug effects—to understand more fully the limitations of their approach than they apparently do at present. This is especially necessary in the area of illicit drugs where, judging from their

183

work, pharmacologists seem to feel that once a drug is outlawed by society they are justified in promoting the reactions of a few individuals into general rules. This approach is very convenient in that it allows them to kill two birds with one stone: to hide the deficiencies of their methodology and to support the laws of their society with "scientific" evidence. Indeed it really gives them three birds, since such judgments almost invariably reflect the moral biases of the judges. In effect, then, in the area of illicit drugs the typical pharmacologist performs a function similar to that of an antivenereal disease film which leaves the powerful impression that celibacy is the wisest course. This is behavior appropriate to preachers but not to anyone posing as a maker of scientific descriptions.

This blurring of roles has consequences more serious than any arising from simple errors on matters of fact. For our body of law is not in theory designed to accommodate the idiosyncracies of individuals, but rather to promote the orderly determination of interests considered common to most members of society. Individual laws and the prevailing preoccupation of law with the protection of property rights may be mistaken, but one cannot imagine a workable body of law capable of doing justice to every individual's wide range of particular needs. The best law can do is to refrain as much as possible from infringing on individual liberties and the expression of individual needs. And any body of work which helps to deprive the individual of his status—as does pharmacology in providing false general rules on the effects of illicit drugs—even before he is subject to the strictures of the law, does a serious disservice to this ideal.

In general, all legislation of morality, whether it be aimed at homosexuals, odd religions, drug users, or any other group which offends the tastes of the majority, tends to unnecessarily deprive individuals of their liberty—and should be questioned by anyone who believes the goal of a free society is to maximize individual liberty. Any law which imposes restrictions in cases where individual liberties do not threaten the

184

liberties of others should be abrogated. This is not always an easy assessment to make, and whether anti-drug legislation is always an unjustified intrusion on individual liberty is a question reasonable citizens can differ on. But what is not debatable is that the use of erroneous data to justify the prohibition of a drug does a disservice to everyone concerned. It permits the jailing of citizens on false grounds and debases the scientific community. It should stop.

Appendices

I

Summary of Arguments Used to Support the Proposition that Cocaine is Not an Addictive, Especially Dangerous Drug

History is written by observers: some are eyewitnesses to the events they describe and interpret, most are not, and none are wholly disinterested. This observer's interest in revealing the absurdity of our drug laws is evident throughout the text. But for those readers who may have lost the arguments used to support this position among the thickets of historical illustration, for students doing book reports, and as a service to overworked reviewers, I present them here in one place.

For a variety of reasons—prominent among which are the limitations of pharmacology to fully ascertain the psychoactive effects of specific drugs, and the misconceptions promulgated by both reasonable and sensationalist authors—cocaine has long been considered an especially dangerous drug. This commonly accepted view has been used to justify harsh penalties for using cocaine, to justify the government's current campaign against cocaine dealers, and to justify the inclusion of cocaine in Schedule II of Title II of the Comprehensive Drug Abuse Prevention and Control Act of 1970. (Listed under Schedule II are those drugs with currently accepted medical use which also have a high potential for abuse and which may lead to severe psychological or physical dependence.)

But the generally accepted findings on the nature of cocaine have changed radically over the years. Cocaine was once considered—and is still considered under most of our statutes—an addictive narcotic drug possessing the typical characteristics of such drugs, namely: the ability to induce physical and psychological dependence; the development of tolerance in the user; and the onset of serious withdrawal symptoms on discontinuation of the drug. Modern researchers, however, all agree (1) that cocaine is not a narcotic drug but a stimulant drug, (2) that physical dependence does not occur, (3) that tolerance does not develop, and (4) that no significant withdrawal symptoms are evident.

The only remaining justification, therefore, for listing cocaine under Schedule II and for the belief that it is an especially dangerous drug is the still generally accepted notion that cocaine use leads to severe psychological dependence: "The *physical* effects of cocaine withdrawal are minor. . . . However, cocaine withdrawal is characterized by a profound psychological manifestation—*depression*—for which cocaine itself appears to the user to be the only remedy. . . . The compulsion to resume cocaine is very strong." The ideas expressed in this quotation are commonly held by researchers who either have not used cocaine themselves or who have not paid proper attention to the reports of those in the best position to know the facts— those who do use cocaine. When they do consult users, they often find the facts to be different from what they had believed. And some of them, including the author just quoted, admit their error and retract their previous statements.

After interviewing some 81 cocaine users and consulting several other investigators, it is clear to me

187

that the psychological depression which almost all current "authorities" insist follows on the discontinuation of cocaine is *not* a condition which any significant number of cocaine users have ever experienced. On the contrary, no "typical" user—that is, one who purchases a gram every two or three weeks—reported experiencing any recognizable discomfort on discontinuing use beyond that which everyone feels when something they like is no longer available. As for that small number of users who take cocaine on a daily basis in either small or relatively large amounts, they do report occasionally experiencing what is often called the "cocaine blues" when they discontinue use. But according to their testimony this is a condition characterized by lassitude, a condition with marked psychological similarities to an alcoholic hangover. It is only very rarely, if ever, a condition analogous to true depression or one which drives them to seek relief in more cocaine. Indeed, cocaine seems to be the last thing anyone wants when feeling this way.

As for there being a strong compulsion to resume cocaine use, this is, as a general statement, devoid of meaning. Some users exhibit such a compulsion, but it doesn't stem from a need to relieve depression. Rather, cocaine being their drug of choice, they procure it whenever they can, finances permitting. The great preponderance of users, however, regard cocaine in a much different way. They like it, and they take it on "special" occasions—in much the same way as those who regularly drink wine with their meals will occasionally treat themselves and their guests to a fine vintage Bordeaux.

Attending to the facts reported by users—as distinguished from what must, given the legal and methodological restrictions under which they operate, be characterized as the speculations of the pharmacologists—there appears no good reason and even less evidence to suggest that cocaine is an especially dangerous drug. The large single doses given for medical reasons have at times produced extremely serious toxic reactions, the doses used in social settings have not. At any rate, a search of the relevant literature fails to show a single case of serious toxic reaction in the past forty years or so.

The conclusion that cocaine is not a dangerous pleasure drug is buttressed by the fact that pure cocaine, when taken in the usual social doses of 20-30 mg repeated every 30 to 60 minutes, and administered in the most common way—by snorting—is not the extremely potent drug it has been made out to be. Rather it is a drug subtle enough that naive users frequently need to have its effects pointed out before they are able to recognize them. Indeed, persons who have thought they were using cocaine but were in fact using highly adulterated cocaine cut with meta-amphetamine (a common street product these days) have on more than one occasion charged a dealer with cheating them after he has sold them high-quality cocaine. They didn't experience the kick they had learned to identify as the kick of cocaine.

II

The Legal Situation

All the data appearing in the following table are current as of June, 1972, except that the California, New York, and Federal provisions are current as of June, 1974. The reader should be aware that in condensing complicated statutes to tabular form, many of the nuances of these statutes are lost. Moreover, state drug laws are frequently amended. Thus anyone wishing to know precisely what the situation in their state is at any given time should check the current status of the laws.

About the table:
  —All sentences are given in years.
  —All fines are given in dollars.
  —In some jurisdictions either a jail sentence, a fine, or both can be meted out. In such cases the phrase "and/or" appears before the fine.
    —The following abbreviations are used:
  NLT = Not less than

NMT = Not more than
NSP = No special provisions for this offense
— = No provision in statute
1 = 1st offense
2 = 2nd offense
S = Subsequent offense

The tables list the penalties for possession and/or sale of cocaine in the 50 states and the District of Columbia. Anyone tried in a Federal District Court faces the following penalty structure:

I *Possession*
    1. NMT 1 yr. and/or $5,000
    S. NMT 2 yrs. and/or $5,000

II *Possession with Intent to Distribute, Distribute, or Sale*
    1. NMT 15 yrs. and/or $25,000
    S. NMT 30 yrs. and/or $50,000

III *Distribution or Sale to Minor*
    1. Twice penalties of II
    S. Three times penalties of II

IV *Persons Engaged in Continuing Criminal Enterprise**
    1. 10 yrs. to life and NMT $100,000
    S. 20 yrs. to life and NMT $200,000

*Essentially those persons identified by narcotics agents as major drug dealers.

STATE	POSSESSION			SALE			SALE TO MINOR		
	NLT (yrs.)	NMT (yrs.)	(Fines) NMT	NLT (yrs.)	NMT (yrs.)	(Fines) NMT	NLT (yrs.)	NMT (yrs.)	(Fines) NMT
Alabama									
1.	2	10	$20,000	5	20	$20,000	10	Life	$20,000
S.	10	40	$20,000	10	40	$20,000	—	—	—
Alaska									
1.	2	10	$5,000	same as possession			10	30	$10,000
2.	10	20	$7,500				15	30	$25,000
S.	20	40	$10,000				Life	—	—
Arizona									
1.	2	10	—	5	15	—	5	10 to Life	—
2.	5	20	—	10	—	—	10	10 to Life	—
S.	15	Life	—	15	—	—	15	15 to Life	—
Arkansas									
1.	2	5	$2,000	same as possession			same as possession		
2.	5	10	$2,000						
S.	10	20	$2,000						
California									
1.	2	10	—	5[1]	15	—	NSP		
2.	5	20	—	10[2]	—	—			
S.	15	Life	—	15[3]	—	—			

1. Must serve NLT 2½ yrs. to be eligible for parole.
2. Must serve NLT 6 yrs. to be eligible for parole.
3. Must serve NLT 15 yrs. to be eligible for parole.

STATE	POSSESSION			SALE			SALE TO MINOR		
	NLT (yrs.)	NMT (yrs.)	(Fines) NMT	NLT (yrs.)	NMT (yrs.)	(Fines) NMT	NLT (yrs.)	NMT (yrs.)	(Fines) NMT
Colorado									
1.	2	15	$10,000	10	20	—		NSP	
2.	5	20	$10,000	15	30	—			
S.	10	30	$10,000	20	40	—			
Connecticut									
1.	—	5 and/or	$ 3,000	5	10	$ 3,000		NSP	
2.	—	15 and/or	$ 5,000	10	15	$ 5,000			
S.	—	25 and/or	$10,000	—	25	—			
Delaware									
1.	—	5	$ 5,000	10	25	$50,000	15	30	court determined
S.	3	10	—	30	99	—	30	99	—
District of Columbia									
1.	—	1 and/or	$ 1,000	same as possession				NSP	
S.	—	10 and/or	$ 5,000						
Florida									
1.	2	5 and/or	$ 5,000	—	10 and/or	$10,000	10	Life	$10,000
2.	5	10 and/or	$10,000	10	20 and/or	$20,000	10	Life	$20,000
S.	10	20 and/or	$20,000	20	Life and/or	$20,000	20	Life	$20,000

STATE	POSSESSION			SALE			SALE TO MINOR		
	NLT (yrs.)	NMT (yrs.)	(Fines) NMT	NLT (yrs.)	NMT (yrs.)	(Fines) NMT	NLT (yrs.)	NMT (yrs.)	(Fines) NMT
Georgia									
1.	2	5	$ 2,000	same as possession				NSP	
2.	5	10	$ 3,000						
S.	10	20	$ 5,000						
Hawaii									
1.	—	1	$ 1,000	—	10	$ 1,000	—	20	$ 1,000
S.	—	1	$ 2,000	—	20	$ 2,000	—	Life	$ 2,000
Idaho									
1.	misdemeanor			—	15 and/or	$25,000	Up to twice the penalty for sale to adult		
S.	misdemeanor			Up to twice the above					
Illinois									
1.	2	10	$ 5,000	10	Life	—		NSP	
S.	5	Life	—	Life	—	—			
Indiana									
1.	2	10	$ 1,000	5	20	$ 2,000		NSP	
S.	5	20	$ 2,000	20	Life	$ 5,000			
Iowa									
1.	2	5	$ 2,000	same as possession			5	20	—
2.	5	10	$ 2,000				5	20	—
S.	10	20	$ 2,000				5	20	—

STATE		POSSESSION			SALE			SALE TO MINOR		
		NLT (yrs.)	NMT (yrs.)	(Fines) NMT	NLT (yrs.)	NMT (yrs.)	(Fines) NMT	NLT (yrs.)	NMT (yrs.)	(Fines) NMT
Kansas	1.	1-3	10	—	same as possession			same as possession		
Kentucky	1.	2	10	$20,000	5	10	$20,000	20	Life	$20,000
	S.	5	20	$20,000	10	40	$20,000			
Louisiana	1.	—	5 and/or	$ 5,000	—	30 and/or	$15,000	Twice penalty for sale to adult		
	S.	—	Twice above	Twice above	—	Twice above				
Maine	1.	2	8	$ 1,000	same as possession			—	20	$10,000
	2.	5	15	$ 2,000						
	S.	10	20	$ 5,000						
Maryland	1.	—	4 and/or	$25,000	—	20	$25,000	NSP		
	S.	—	—		—	Twice above				
Massachusetts	1.	—	3½	$ 1,000	5	10	—	20	25	—
	S.	—	—	—	10	25	—	20	50 and no probation or parole	—
Michigan	1.	—	10	$ 5,000	20	Life	—	NSP		
	2.	—	20	$ 5,000						
	S.	20	40	$ 5,000						

STATE	POSSESSION			SALE			SALE TO MINOR		
	NLT (yrs.)	NMT (yrs.)	(Fines) NMT	NLT (yrs.)	NMT (yrs.)	(Fines) NMT	NLT (yrs.)	NMT (yrs.)	(Fines) NMT
Minnesota									
1.	5	20	$10,000	same as possession			10	40	$20,000
Mississippi									
1.	—	6 and/or	$ 2,000	same as possession			—	12 and/or	$ 2,000
Missouri									
1.	½	20 and/or	$ 2,000	5	Life		Death		
2.	5	Life	—	10	Life				
S.	10	Life	—						
Montana									
1.	—	5	—	1	Life	—			
Nebraska									
1.	2	5	$ 3,000	same as possession				NSP	
2.	5	10	$ 5,000						
S.	10	20	$ 5,000						
Nevada									
1.	1	6	$ 2,000	1	20 (no parole)	$ 5,000	Life	(parole after 7 yrs.)	
2.	1	10	$ 2,000	Life		$ 5,000	Life	(no parole)	
S.	1	20	$ 5,000						
New Hampshire									
1.	—	5 and/or	$ 2,000	—	20 and/or	$ 5,000		NSP	
S.	—	10 and/or	$ 5,000	—	25				

STATE	POSSESSION NLT (yrs.)	NMT (yrs.)	(Fines) NMT	SALE NLT (yrs.)	NMT (yrs.)	(Fines) NMT	SALE TO MINOR NLT (yrs.)	NMT (yrs.)	(Fines) NMT
New Jersey 1.	—	5	and/or $15,000	—	12 and/or	$25,000	—	Twice penalty for	
S.		Twice above			Twice above			sale to adult	
New York									
I Less than ⅛ oz.	—	1	$ 1,000	1-8 ⅓*	Life	—		NSP	
II Less than 1 oz.	one-half 9-25 actual max. set by court		—	6-8 ⅓*	Life	—			
III Less than 2 oz.	6-8 ⅓* Life		—	15-25*	Life	—			
IV 2 oz. or more	15-25* Life		—						

*Minimum of mandatory life sentences, all of which carry lifetime parole provisions.

STATE	POSSESSION NLT (yrs.)	NMT (yrs.)	(Fines) NMT	SALE NLT (yrs.)	NMT (yrs.)	(Fines) NMT	SALE TO MINOR NLT (yrs.)	NMT (yrs.)	(Fines) NMT
N. Carolina 1.	—	5 and/or	$ 1,000		same as possession		10	20	—
2.	5	10 and/or	$ 2,000				—	—	—
S.	15	Life	$ 3,000						
N. Dakota 1.	—	5 and/or	$ 2,500	—	20 and/or	$10,000	—	40 and/or	$20,000
S.	—	10 and/or	$ 5,000	—	40 and/or	$20,000		Twice above	

STATE	POSSESSION			SALE			SALE TO MINOR		
	NLT (yrs.)	NMT (yrs.)	(Fines) NMT	NLT (yrs.)	NMT (yrs.)	(Fines) NMT	NLT (yrs.)	NMT (yrs.)	(Fines) NMT
Ohio*				20	40	—	30	Life	—
1.	2	5	$10,000			—			—
2.	5	10	$10,000						
S.	10	20	$10,000						

* Also has special provisions for "possession for sale":

	NLT	NMT	
1.	10	20	—
2.	15	30	—
S.	20	40	—

(Other offenses: Carnal knowledge of another person, knowing that such person is under the influence of a narcotic drug—and cocaine is a narcotic drug under Ohio statutes—is punishable as follows:

1. 2-15 and NMT $10,000
2. 5-20 and NMT $10,000
S. 10-30 and NMT $10,000

STATE	POSSESSION			SALE	SALE TO MINOR
Oklahoma				same as possession	NSP
1.	—	5 and/or	$ 1,000		
2.	5	10 and/or	$ 3,000		
S.	10	20 and/or	$ 5,000		
Oregon				same as possession	NSP
1.	—	10 and/or	$10,000		

STATE	POSSESSION			SALE			SALE TO MINOR		
	NLT (yrs.)	NMT (yrs.)	(Fines) NMT	NLT (yrs.)	NMT (yrs.)	(Fines) NMT	NLT (yrs.)	NMT (yrs.)	(Fines) NMT
Pennsylvania									
1.	2	5	$ 2,000	5	20	$ 5,000		NSP	
2.	5	10	$ 5,000	10	30	$15,000			
S.	10	30	$ 7,500	Life	—	$30,000			
Rhode Island*									
1.	2	15	$10,000	20	40	—	30	Life	—
2.	5	20	$10,000	—	—	—	—	—	—
S.	10	30	$10,000	—	—	—	—	—	—
* Also has special provision for "possession for sale":									
1.	10	20	—						
2.	15	30	—						
S.	20	40							
S. Carolina									
1.	—	2 and/or	$ 2,000	—	3½ and/or	$ 3,500	—	5 and/or	$ 5,000
2.	2	5 and/or	$ 5,000	—	5	—	—	10	—
S.	10	20	—	—	10	—			
S. Dakota									
1.	—	5 and/or	$ 5,000	same as possession			Twice penalty for sale		
2.	—	15 and/or	$15,000						
S.	—	40 and/or	$20,000						

STATE	POSSESSION			SALE			SALE TO MINOR		
	NLT (yrs.)	NMT (yrs.)	(Fines) NMT	NLT (yrs.)	NMT (yrs.)	(Fines) NMT	NLT (yrs.)	NMT (yrs.)	(Fines) NMT
Tennessee									
1.	2	5	$ 500		same as possession			NSP	
2.	5	10	$ 500						
S.	10	20	$ 500						
Texas									
1.	2	Life	—	5	Life	—	5	Life	—
S.	10	Life	—	10	Life	—	10	Life and possible death	—
Utah									
1.	—	½ and/or	$ 299	—	15 and/or	$15,000	—	20 and/or	$15,000
2.	—	1 and/or	$ 1,000	7½	—	—	10	—	—
S.	—	5	—						
Vermont									
Less than 1 oz.	—	1 and/or	$ 1,000	1.	5 and/or	$10,000		NSP	
1 oz. or more	—	5 and/or	$ 5,000	S. 10	25	$25,000			
Virginia									
1.	1	10	—	1	40 and/or	$25,000	5	40 and/or	$50,000
S.	1	20	$10,000	10	Life and/or	$50,000	—	—	—
Washington									
1.	5	20 and/or	$10,000		same as possession		20	40	$50,000
2.	10	20 and/or	$10,000				—	—	—
S.	15	40 and/or	$25,000						

STATE	POSSESSION			SALE			SALE TO MINOR		
	NLT (yrs.)	NMT (yrs.)	(Fines) NMT	NLT (yrs.)	NMT (yrs.)	(Fines) NMT	NLT (yrs.)	NMT (yrs.)	(Fines) NMT
West Virginia	¼	½ and/or $ 1,000	Twice above	1	15 and/or $25,000	Twice above	2	30 and/or $25,000	Twice above
Wisconsin									
1.	—	1 and/or $ 500		—	5 and/or $ 5,000		—	15	
2.	—	2 and/or $ 1,000		—	10 and/or $10,000		30	Life	
S.	—	—		—	—		Life	—	
Wyoming									
1.	—	½ and/or $ 1,000		—	20 and/or $25,000		Twice penalty for sale to adult		
2.	—	½ and/or $ 1,000		—	40 and/or $50,000				
S.	—	5 and/or $ 5,000		—	—				

III

Do Our Drug Laws Discourage the Use of Illicit Drugs?

I have argued that cocaine is not an especially dangerous drug and have stated my belief that the prohibition against cocaine (and other illicit drugs) should be abolished. At the same time I recognize that even if one agrees cocaine is not especially dangerous, one may still believe that its use should be discouraged and that prison sentences for the apprehended sellers and users of cocaine will act as a deterrent to others. The question then is whether prison sentences act as an effective deterrent in drug cases. The answer is no.

An examination of the historical record makes it abundantly clear that despite a continuing escalation of the penalties for possessing, using, and selling illicit drugs, the traffic in them has continually increased rather than declined. This state of affairs has led advocates of still heavier sanctions to argue that if the police were given more leeway and the judges more power, the certainty of apprehension and subsequent conviction would be increased and thus the deterrent

202

effect of the laws increased; or, at the very least, that harsher penalties would be a powerful deterrent in and of themselves.

Such arguments were given by those favoring passage of New York state's current drug law, the most severe in the nation. But this law has been in effect since September 1, 1973, and to date its effects have been precisely those predicted by the district attorneys of the state, the large majority of whom opposed the law: arrests and convictions are at an all-time low, while the drug traffic continues to thrive. There are probably a number of reasons for this, and three likely ones are that the prospect of arresting a dealer who faces no greater sentence for murder than he does for selling drugs has greatly disheartened honest narcotics officers; the severity of the penalties encourages greater corruption among dishonest officers; and grand juries have been loathe to indict and juries to convict in the face of such penalties.

In general, the history of our drug laws provides little reason and less evidence to suggest that the current federal and state laws deter the sale and use of illicit drugs, or that harsher laws will do so. The difficulty of making arrests and procuring convictions in situations where the offence is between consenting parties is legendary, and thus the factor which is generally considered the prime deterrent factor—a high degree of certainty of arrest and conviction—is lacking. Unless we are willing to advocate the imposition of a full-blown police state there is no reason to believe that any considerable degree of certainty can be achieved. Indeed certainty is not guaranteed even then. In the Soviet Union, a police state par excellence, the incidence of illicit drug use has risen to the point where it is now an officially recognized problem.

To conclude, the common experience of mankind has demonstrated the impossibility of effectively prohibiting what any significant number of people wish to do in the privacy of their own homes. The ineffectiveness of a whole series of laws proscribing certain sexual acts, the total failure of the prohibition against alcohol, and the constant rise in the use of illicit drugs despite ever-increasing penalties all testify to this. As matters now stand, the drug laws can be enforced in only an extremely discriminatory way—i.e., by the apprehension of a miniscule percentage of offenders. Since their fate does not deter others, justice is not served.

IV

The Refining of Cocaine

The process can be separated into three stages: from coca leaves to crude cocaine, from crude cocaine to rock, and from rock to flake. The first two are essential to the production of usable cocaine, the third is a cleaning-up procedure employed to obtain a purer form of cocaine.

Reducing coca to crude cocaine is usually done near the growing areas. Vats holding from one to 15 tons of leaves are commonly used. Depending on the cocaine content of the leaves, a ton of coca will yield from 15 to 20 pounds of cocaine.

First Stage

a. The vat is filled with powdered coca leaves. Dilute sulphuric acid (water and sulphuric acid) is added to leach out the cocaine and associated alkaloids.
b. Sodium carbonate is added to make the solution

alkaline and to precipitate the cocaine and associated alkaloids in solid form.

c. A light petroleum such as benzene is added to the solution, which is then stirred. The benzene takes up the cocaine and other alkaloids.

d. The benzene solution is then drawn off and washed with water to remove the last traces of sulphuric acid. (In an alkaline solution, cocaine is indissoluble in water, and thus none is lost in this process.)

e. The washed solution is again treated with dilute sulphuric acid and stirred violently for 30 to 40 minutes to redissolve the cocaine.

f. After standing a short while, the cocaine and associated alkaloids (all of which are suspended in the dilute sulphuric acid solution) are drawn off, leaving the benzene to be used again.

g. This acid solution is treated with sodium carbonate to precipitate the cocaine and allowed to stand for 12 hours.

h. It is then passed through a filter which collects the precipitate.

i. The precipitate, cocaine and associated alkaloids, is washed with distilled water to remove the acid and pressed into a paste.

This brownish paste is crude cocaine and, since it neither dissolves readily in water nor passes through the mucous membranes, is of no value medicinally or socially. The product used in both these situations is cocaine hydrochloride, and is obtained as follows:

Second Stage

a. The crude cocaine is dissolved in dilute hydrochloric acid (water and hydrochloric acid).

b. It is then treated with a solution of potassium permanganate, which destroys the associated alkaloids before attacking the cocaine.

c. The action of the potassium permanganate is checked by the addition of sodium carbonate, which also precipitates the cocaine in solid form.

d. The solution is passed through a filter which collects the cocaine.

e. As the cocaine dries, it tends to cake, forming rock cocaine.

At this point, the rock cocaine product is a minimum of 70 per cent pure and may be as high as 86 per cent pure. Most illicit cocaine is in rock form (or powder, pulverized rock). To obtain flake cocaine, which is the pharmaceutical, and finest available illicit, variety, additional steps are required:

Third Stage

a. The rock is pulverized.

b. It is then dissolved in an alkaline water solution.

c. Petroleum ether or benzene is added to take up the cocaine.

d. Methanol and hydrochloric acid are added to precipitate the cocaine in solid form.

e. The solution is passed through a filter which collects the cocaine.

The cocaine is now relatively pure and may remain in crystals (flakes) rather than caking as it dries. The more often the third stage is repeated the purer the cocaine obtained. Pharmaceutical cocaine is a minimum 99 per cent pure, and illicit flake cocaine has been tested as high as 95 per cent pure.

The refining procedures outlined above are not the only way of obtaining cocaine from coca. Many variations are employed, the specific details of which are kept as trade secrets by the manufacturers. The general methods, however, are all similar—as the following process for preparing cocaine on a small scale illustrates:

"One hundred grammes of finely ground leaves are moistened with 100 c.c. of 7 per cent solution of sodium carbonate, packed in a percolator, and sufficient kerosene added to make 700 c.c. of percolate. This is transferred to a separator, and 30 c.c. of 2 per cent solution of hydrochloric acid added and shaken. After separation the watery solution is drawn off from below into a smaller separator, and this process is repeated three times, the alkaloid being in the smaller separator as an acid hydrochlorate. This is precipitated in ether with sodium carbonate, and evaporated at low heat with constant stirring. . . ."*

*W. G. Mortimer, *Peru: History of Coca, "The Divine Plant" of the Incas* (New York: J. H. Vail and Company, 1901) pp. 311-312.

V

Storing Cocaine

The pharmacological texts all advise that cocaine be stored in "well-closed, light-resistant containers."

Cocaine folklore agrees with this and, in addition, has perpetuated the beliefs that (a) refrigeration prolongs potency, and that (b) the various cuts used to adulterate cocaine decrease the potency of the remaining cocaine over a period of time.

The facts are somewhat different. A well-closed container is all that is necessary to preserve the potency of cocaine. (Water dissolves cocaine and water is present in air.) The texts recommend a light-resistant container because this is standard practice in storing drugs, but it would take several years of exposure to sunlight to measurably affect cocaine's potency. Refrigeration is also unnecessary. Pharmaceutical cocaine was still 98 per cent pure after standing on a shelf for four years, according to a Drug Enforcement Agency chemist. The assertion that various cuts reduce potency over a period of time is not true. Cocaine is a very stable compound, and none of the known cuts affect it. What percentage of cocaine is present after cutting remains present. Apart from exposure to air, about the only way potency can be reduced over a short period of time is when the refining process has been sloppy and all the sodium carbonate has not been removed.

VI

Signs of, and Treatment for, Acute Toxic Reactions

Though acute toxic reactions are very rare, the initial indications of too great an intake of cocaine are insomnia, anxiety, undue aggressiveness, unwarranted impatience, impotency, tender and irritated nostrils, nosebleeds, pallor, cold sweats, and a feeling of heaviness throughout the limbs.

Any user who notes any of these signs should lay off the cocaine. Continued usage may lead to acute toxic reactions, the symptoms of which are as follows:

Stage	Central Nervous System	Cardiovascular & Circulatory System	Respiratory System
Initial	Fainting, Convulsions.	Increased pulse rate and increased blood pressure.	Rapid, shallow breathing. Blue skin color.
Secondary	Muscular paralysis. Loss of reflexes. Unconsciousness. Loss of vital functions. Death.	Circulatory collapse. No detectable pulse. Cardiovascular collapse. Death.	Respiratory failure. Ashen gray skin color. Death.

The progression from excessive stimulation to depression and from the first signs of depression to death usually occur very rapidly—so rapidly that if an overdose has been taken in any setting other than a medical one it is unlikely that the victim will survive long enough to receive treatment. Treatment, therefore, should begin as soon as there is any indication of an acute toxic reaction. That is, as soon as any of the symptoms of the initial stage are noted.

The following procedures have been recommended, the first two steps of which may be administered by laymen until expert professional help arrives:

1. Administration of oxygen: by positive pressure and artificial respiration if necessary. Be certain that an open airway is present.

2. Trendelenburg position (head down). Wrap arms and legs if necessary to increase central return of blood.

3. Inject small amounts of short-acting barbiturates (e.g., 25-50 mg. sodium pentothal) *if* convulsions are present. May be repeated, but *gently*. (Do *not* force general depressant effect to point of no return.)

4. Administer intravenous stimulants for cardiotonic effect (e.g., 10-20 mg. phenylephrine).

5. Keep patient cool, and keep crowds away.

6. General muscle relaxants may be given (e.g., curare, succinylcholine) to facilitate administration of positive pressure oxygen.

7. Continuously monitor vital signs.

VII

Additional Methods of Determining the Purity of Cocaine

Those with access to simple laboratory equipment may consult standard texts such as the *United States Dispensary* for methods of determining the purity of cocaine. For those who do not, and who are not satisfied by the tests described in Chapter VII, the following may be used:

(1) *The Cobalt Test*: A commercially marketed test sold in many of the shops which cater to illicit drug users. It is a simple procedure, the intensity of the blue resulting from the mixing of cocaine and cobalt indicating the purity of the sample. Directions come with the kit.

(2) *The Methanol Test*: With the exception of the synthetic local anesthetics such as procaine and the amphetamines such as methedrine, the common cutting agents do not dissolve in methanol (pure alcohol), whereas cocaine does. Therefore if you (1) measure out two small and equal portions of a sample, (2) place them in two teaspoons, (3) add one-quarter of

a teaspoon of methanol to one of the measures, and (4) stir mixture thoroughly—anything which remains undissolved is not cocaine. You then compare the remaining material with the untouched measure to determine the amount of cut and/or impurities in the sample. If the tested measure holds, for example, 50 per cent as much material as the untested measure, the sample cannot be more than 50 per cent pure. But since the synthetic local anesthetics and methedrine do dissolve in methanol, there is no assurance that the sample is 50 per cent pure cocaine. Some of the dissolved material may be one of these cuts.

If other tests have indicated the presence of procaine or a similar synthetic, any light petroleum mixed in a sodium bicarbonate solution can be added to the measure in place of methanol. This will dissolve the cocaine but not the suspected cut and anything that remains will be the cut.

(3) *Volume Differentiation*: This is a relatively crude test and not practicable when applied to quantities of less than one-half ounce. Greater accuracy will be attained with quantities of one ounce and over. The underlying principle of the volume differentiation test is that pure cocaine weighs less in equal volume than any of the generally used cuts. Thus the larger the volume for a given weight, the purer the cocaine. A typical 86 per cent pure ounce will measure 50 level one-quarter teaspoons. If cut, there will be less than 50 one-quarter teaspoons even though the weight is precisely the same.

Since different cuts have different weight-volume ratios, this test cannot provide the precise amount of cut. It only indicates the gross presence of a cut and a rough approximation of the amount of cut.

VIII

Weights and Measures

The most common retail quantities of cocaine are the "spoon" and the gram. A gram is a gram, but a spoon may vary anywhere from one-sixteenth to one-half of a measuring teaspoon. There is then no standard spoon, but the "accepted" spoon quantity is one-quarter of a measuring teaspoon.

1 spoon	=	¼ measuring tsp or .56 grams
1 gram	=	approximately ½ measuring teaspoon; or 15.4 grains
¼ ounce	=	7 grams
½ ounce	=	14 grams
1 ounce ("piece", "zee")	=	28.35 grams
⅛ kilogram ("eighth")	=	4 ounces + 13 grams; or 125 grams
¼ kilogram ("quarter")	=	8 ounces + 26 grams; or 250 grams

½ kilogram ("half")	= 17 ounces + 24 grams; or 1 lb., 1.9 ounces; or 500 grams
1 kilogram ("kee")	= 35 ounces + 20 grams; or 2 lbs., 3.2 ounces; or 1,000 grams

IX

A Cocaine Chronology

?—9th Cent. A.D.   The pre-Inca period. Yunga tribe
legend relates how tribe finds and sustains itself
on coca after being driven into the high mountains by the god Khunu.

10th—12th Cent.   Trepanned skulls from this period
found in Andes tombs, and evidence strongly
suggests that the cocaine-bearing juice of the coca
leaf was used as a local anesthetic in these operations.

13th—16th Cent.   The Inca Empire. Unlike the Yunga
legend, the Inca legends maintain that coca was
a gift of the Sun God, Manco Capac. Inca attempt
to keep coca for themselves, but long before the
arrival of Pizarro coca is being used by all classes.

15th—16th Cent.   The great age of exploration which
brought coffee, tea, tobacco, opium, and coca to
Europe.

1531—1536   Pizarro arrives in Peru and conquers
Inca. Spanish, believing that coca-chew~ ~ is an

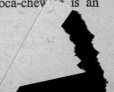

idle and expensive luxury and its effects either imaginary or the product of a pact with the devil, try to prohibit use of coca.

1550 By this date at the latest—since the church is now being largely supported by a tithe on coca—the Spaniards, faced with Indians who won't work the gold and silver mines without their daily coca, have retracted the prohibition.

1550 or 1553 Pedro Cieza de Leon publishes *Chronica del Peru* in which he records the history of the Inca and gives descriptions of coca and its use. He believes its effects are either imaginary or the result of a pact with devil.

1565 Nicolas Monardes, drawing chiefly on the work of Cieza, publishes first European book on coca.

1590 Joseph de Acosta, a Jesuit priest, publishes *Natural History of the Indies* in which he declares the effects of coca are real, not imaginary.

1609 Garcilasso de la Vega publishes *Royal Commentaries of the Incas,* a history which includes detailed account of coca from planting to preparation of the leaf for chewing. Attempts to convince Europeans that the effects of coca are real.

17th—18th Cent. Coca elicits little interest from Europeans, probably because most imported coca has lost its potency during the long voyage.

1783 A. L. de Jussieu classes coca with the genus erythroxylon.

1838 Swiss naturalist Von Tschudi visits Andes region, chews coca, and writes enthusiastically about its benefits.

1855 Probable date when Gaedecke first isolates coca's chief alkaloid and names it erythroxyline.

1859 Dr. Paolo Mantegazza publishes essay praising coca's ability to lessen fatigue, stimulate strength, elevate the spirits, and support potency and sexual desire.

1859 or 1860 Albert Niemann independently isolates chief alkaloid of coca and names it cocaine.

1862 Schroff, a German medical researcher, notes that cocaine numbs the tongue.

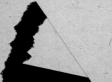

1863 or 1865   Angelo Mariani introduces "Vin Mariani," a preparation of coca and wine which is destined to become immensely popular.

1868   A Peruvian physician, Thomas Moreno y Maiz, suggests that cocaine might be a useful local anesthetic.

1878   An American, Dr. W. H. Bentley, announces that cocaine is useful in treating morphine addiction.

1880—1882   American medical journals carry many articles on cocaine's efficacy in treating morphine addiction.

1883   German army physician, Dr. Theodor Aschenbrandt, issues cocaine to troops and reports they exhibit more energy and less fatigue than those who didn't have it.

1884   Sigmund Freud publishes *Uber Coca,* in which he describes effects of cocaine on himself and others. He is enthusiastic about its euphoric stimulant properties, and suggests several other medical uses for it—among them local anesthesia. His methodology in testing and describing effects makes him founder of psychopharmacology.

1884   Carl Koller follows his friend Freud's suggestion and demonstrates cocaine's usefulness as a local anesthetic in eye surgery.

1884   Dr. William Stewart Halsted of New York injects cocaine into a nerve trunk and obtains anesthesia of all areas served by the trunk.

1884—1885   Following Koller's demonstration, medical community becomes enthusiastic about cocaine. It becomes new wonder drug, patent medicine manufacturers exploit it, and the pleasure-use of cocaine grows rapidly.

1885   Dr. J. Leonard Corning of New York suggests cocaine for spinal anesthesia.

1885—1887   Freud attacked by addiction specialists for maintaining that cocaine is useful in withdrawing addicts from morphine. He is accused of releasing the "third scourge of mankind" (after alcohol and opium). Cocaine is denounced as an addictive drug worse than morphine.

1885   John Styth Pemberton of Atlanta, Georgia, introduces "French Wine Coca—Ideal Nerve and Tonic Stimulant" to compete with "Vin Mariani."

1886   Pemberton introduces "Coca-Cola," a soft-drink syrup based on cocaine and caffeine—the forerunner of dozens of cocaine-based "soft" drinks.

1886   Sir Arthur Conan Doyle gives publicity to cocaine when he has Sherlock Holmes use it in "A Scandal in Bohemia." He confuses cocaine's effects, however, with those of morphine.

1888   Conan Doyle, in *The Sign of the Four* demonstrates he understands the true effects of cocaine.

1885—1906   American patent medicine industry spreads cocaine all over the country in hundreds of tonics, cold "cures," asthma "cures," addiction "cures," and the like.

1887—1914   Forty-six states pass laws to regulate the use and distribution of cocaine, whereas only twenty-nine states pass such laws against the opiates.

1898—1914   Concerted campaign to link the use of cocaine with blacks, the poor, and criminals.

1903   Coca-Cola, under pressure from Southern politicians, takes cocaine out of Coca-Cola.

1906   Pure Food and Drug Act requiring contents to be listed on label effectively eliminates cocaine from most patent medicines and soft drinks.

1914   First federal antidrug law, the Harrison Act, treats cocaine as an especially dangerous drug, providing greater restrictions for it than for the opiates.

1914—1930   More cocaine used in America than ever before even though its legal distribution is greatly curtailed and illicit prices rise continually. Europe, particularly Germany, France, and England, much concerned about the spread of cocaine use.

1916   England passes strict anticocaine law four years before restricting use of the opiates.

1922   Amendment to Narcotic Drugs Import and Export Act clearly and mistakenly identifies cocaine as a "narcotic"—a deliberate misclassification perpetuated in the Comprehensive Drug Abuse Prevention and Control Act of 1970.

1930—mid 1960s Cocaine very much underground. Use confined to very limited areas.

1932 Amphetamines marketed. As a far cheaper, longer lasting rough analog to cocaine, they insure its continuing demise. Amphetamines and meta-amphetamines (speed) keep increasing in popularity among counterculture people until around 1966.

1967—1969 Speed considered a "bad" drug by illicit users, and cocaine starts making a comeback.

1970—1972 The new boom years for cocaine. Spreads through both counterculture and "straight" circles. The "in" drug of rock, television, advertising, etc. Used by the whole cross-section of affluent Americans.

1972—1974 As a result of organized crime elements, chiefly Cubans, moving in on areas hitherto controlled by white middle-class dealers, the price of illicit cocaine doubles. In New York, the ounce that sold for $900 in 1972 brings $2,000 in 1974. Pure cocaine is hard to find along the Eastern seaboard unless buyer deals in kilo lots. Law enforcement agencies devote 50 per cent of their resources to combating cocaine traffic.

Selected Bibliography

On Coca and Cocaine:

W. G. Mortimer, *Peru History of Coça, "The Divine Plant" of the Incas* (New York: J. H. Vail and Co., 1901) The classic work on the history of coca.

Richard Woodley, *Dealer, Portrait of a Cocaine Merchant* (New York: Warner Paperback Library, 1972) The best study of a dealer, and dealing, I have read.

James H. Woods and David A. Downs, "The Psychopharmacology of Cocaine," *Drug Use in America: Problem in Perspective, The Technical Papers of the Second Report of the National Commission on Marihuana and Drug Abuse,* Volume I, March, 1973, pp. 116-139. A careful review of the relevant medical literature.

Cocaine Papers (New York: Stonehill Publishing Co., 1974) New translations of Freud's five papers and essays by several contributors on the general subject. Thoroughly academic.

On the History of American Drug Laws:

Richard J. Bonnie and Charles H. Whitebread, II, "The Forbidden Fruit and the Tree of Knowledge: An Inquiry into the Legal History of American Marijuana Prohibition," *56 Virginia Law Review,* October, 1970, pp. 971-1203.
  Anyone wishing to know how we got the drug laws we have, couldn't do better than to read this. A first-rate piece of work.

Gerald T. McLaughlin, "Cocaine: The History and Regulation of a Dangerous Drug," *58 Cornell Law Review,* March, 1973, pp. 537-573.
  Part I, *The Drug,* is sketchy, but Part II, *History of Federal and State Legislation,* is useful.

Specific and general drug studies which, in my opinion, are the best of their kind; and which offer the reader well-considered views on the relation between drugs, politics, the law, and society:

Richard Ashley, *Heroin, The Myths and the Facts* (New York: St. Martin's Press, 1972)

Edward Brecher and the Editors of Consumer Reports, *Licit & Illicit Drugs,* The Consumers Union Report on Narcotics, Stimulants, Depressants, Inhalants, Hallucinogens, and Marijuana—including Caffeine, Nicotine, and Alcohol (Boston: Little, Brown and Company, 1972)

John Kaplan, *Marihuana—The New Prohibition* (New York: World, 1970)

Rufus King, *The Drug Hang-up: America's Fifty Folly* (New York: W. W. Norton, 1972)

Alfred R. Lindesmith, *The Addict and the Law* (New York: Vintage Books, 1965)

Alfred McCoy, *The Politics of Heroin in South East Asia* (New York: Harper and Row, 1972)

David Musto, *The American Disease, Origins of Narcotic Control* (New Haven: Yale University Press, 1973)

Charles Perry and Mildred Pellens, *The Opium Problem* (New York Committee on Drug Addictions, Bureau of Social Hygiene, Inc., 1928)

Norman E. Zinberg and John A. Robertson, *Drugs and the Public* (New York: Simon & Schuster, 1972)

Andrew Weil, *The Natural Mind,* A New Way of Looking at Drugs and the Higher Consciousness (Boston: Houghton Mifflin Company, 1972)

Footnotes

Preface

1. Rufus King, *62 Yale Law Journal*, 1953.

Chapter 1

1. Andrew T. Weil, "Altered States of Consciousness," in *Dealing with Drug Abuse, A Report to the Ford Foundation* (New York: Praeger Publishers, 1972), p. 339.
2. For example, see Anthony Trollope's *The Three Clerks* where cigars and gin compete as symbols of debauchery.
3. Louis Lewin, quoted in R. S. DeRopp, *Drugs and the Mind* (New York: Grove Press, Inc., 1961), p. 276.
4. W. G. Mortimer, *Peru History of Coca, "The Divine Plant" of the Incas* (New York: J. H. Vail and Com-

. See Chapter VI.
6. *Mortimer*, p. 149 says 1550 and Norman Taylor, *Plant Drugs That Changed the World* (New York: Dodd, Mead & Company, 1965), p. 6 says 1553.
7. *Mortimer*, p. 160.
8. Ibid., p. 168.
9. William H. Hodge, "Coca," in *Natural History*, February, 1947, p. 87.
10. Norman Taylor, op. cit., p. 11.
11. *Mortimer*, p. 162.
12. Ibid., 171.
13. Paolo Mantegazza, *Sulle virtu ignieiche e medicinali della coca*, Milan, 1859.
14. Quoted in *Mortimer*, p. 177.
15. *Mortimer*, pp. 16, 17.
16. Marcel Granier-Doyeux, "From Opium to LSD, The Long History of Drugs," *21 UNESCO Courier*, May, 1968, p. 11.
17. Garcilasso de la Vega, cited in Sigmund Freud, *"Uber Coca," The Cocaine Papers* (Vienna: Dunguin Press, 1963).
18. *Mortimer*, p. 20.
19. Ibid., p. 152.
20. Hector P. Blejer, "Coca Leaf and Cocaine Addiction—Some Historical Notes," *Canadian Medical Association Journal*, 93, September 25, 1965, p. 701.
21. Garcilasso de la Vega, op. cit.
22. *Mortimer*, p. 20.
23. Ibid., p. 157.
24. Ibid., p. 160
25. Norman, Taylor, *Narcotics: Nature's Dangerous Gifts*, 1966, p. 65 (15,000,000); Joel Fort, *The Pleasure Seekers*, 1969, p. 41 (10,000,000); Richard Woodley, *Dealer, Portrait of a Cocaine Merchant*, p. 49 (8,000,000); and Richard R. Lingeman, *Drugs From A to Z: A Dictionary*, p. 43 (90 percent).
26. See, e.g., "Report of the International Narcotics Control Board on its work in 1970," United Nations, *Bulletin On Narcotics*, Vol. XXIII, No. 3, July—September 1971, pp. 33-36.

27. Edward Brecher, *Licit & Illicit Drugs,* (Boston: Little, Brown and Company, 1972), p. 48.

28. Gerald T. McLaughlin, "Cocaine: The History and Regulation of a Dangerous Drug," *58 Cornell Law Review,* March, 1973, p. 542.

29. See *Bulletin on Narcotics,* Vol XXIII, op. cit. and any current reports of the International Narcotics Control Board, such as in *Bulletin on Narcotics,* Vol. XXV, No. 2, 1973.

30. See C. Gutierrez-Noriega and V. Z. Ortiz, *Estudios sobre la Coca y la Cocaine en el Peru,* Lima, 1947; C. Gutierrez-Noriega and V. W. Von Hagen, "The Strange Case of the Coca Leaf," 70 *Scientific Monthly,* 1950, pp. 81-89; and J. C. Negrette and H. B. M. Murphy, "Psychological deficit in chewers of coca leaf," United Nations, *Bulletin on Narcotics,* Vol. IXX, 1967, pp. 11-18.

31. Ibid. and Granier-Doyeux, op. cit., p. 12.

32. Granier-Doyeux, op. cit., p. 12.

33. Ibid., p. 12, and footnote 30.

34. Norman Taylor, *Plant Drugs That Changed the World,* op. cit., p. 9.

35. Edward Brecher, op. cit., p. 271.

36. Ibid.

37. Granier-Doyeux, op. cit., p. 12.

38. See, e.g., H. A. Abramson (ed.), *The Use of LSD in Psychotherapy and Alcoholism* (Indianapolis: Bobbs-Merrill Co., Inc., 1967).

39. There are over 200 varieties of the genus Erythroxylon. (C.F. David J. Rogers, "Divine" Leaves of the Incas, *Natural History,* January, 1963, p. 33) and see *Mortimer,* Chapter VIII for an extensive discussion of the many varieties of Erythroxylon coca.

40. *Mortimer,* pp. 233-235.

41. *Mortimer,* p. 254; William Alfred Reid, "Coca" in *Commodities of Commerce Series No. 20,* Washington, 1920; and T. A. Henry, *The Plant Alkaloids* (Philadelphia: P. Blakiston's Son & Co., 1924), p. 94.

42. *Mortimer,* p. 240.

43. Ibid., p. 241.

44. *Statistics on Narcotic Drugs for 1970* (New York: United Nations, 1971).

45. *Mortimer,* p. 249.

46. Ibid.
47. E.g., *National Clearinghouse for Drug Abuse Information,* Report Series 11, No. 1, *Cocaine,* January, 1972, p. 3.
48. Granier-Doyeux, op. cit., p. 12.
49. C.F. Norman Taylor, *Plant Drugs That Changed the World,* op. cit., p. 16; Richard R. Lingeman, *Drugs from A to Z: A Dictionary,* op. cit., p. 43; and McLaughlin, op. cit., p. 543 to name a few.
50. See Chapter VIII.
51. Charles Perry, "The Star-Spangled Powder, or Through History with Coke-Spoon and Nasal Spray," *Rolling Stone,* Issue No. 115, August 17, 1972.

Chapter II

1. G. M. Hocking, "Alkaloids," in *Collier's Encyclopedia,* Vol. 8, (New York: Crowell-Collier Educational Corp., 1968), p. 564.
2. Ibid.
3. Norman Taylor, *Plant Drugs That Changed the World* (New York: Dodd, Mead & Company, 1965), p. 212.
4. G. M. Hocking, op. cit., p. 565.
5. Norman Taylor, op. cit., p. 213.
6. D. W. Maurer & V. H. Vogel, *Narcotics and Narcotic Addiction* (3rd ed.; Springfield: Charles C. Thomas, 1967), pp. 133-134; and *Remington's Pharmaceutical Sciences* (4th ed.; Easton, Pa.: Mack Publishing Co., 1970), p. 1067.
7. H. K. Becker, "Carl Koller and Cocaine, "The *Psychoanalytic Quarterly,* Vol. 32, No. 3, 1963, p. 323; W. G. Mortimer, *Peru History of Coca,* "The *Divine Plant of the Incas* (New York: Vail and Company, 1901), p. 295; Norman Taylor, *Plant Drugs That Changed the World* (New York: Dodd, Mead & Company, 1965), p. 14; J. H. Woods and D. A. Downs "The Psychopharmacology of Cocaine," in *Drug use in America: problem in perspective, The Technical Papers of the Second Report of the National Commission on Marihuana and Drug Abuse*

(Washington, D.C.: U. S. Government Printing Office, March, 1973), p. 117.

8. Richard H. Blum & Associates, *Drugs I: Society and Drugs* (San Francisco: Jossey-Blass, Inc., 1970), p. 102; *National Clearinghouse for Drug Abuse Information*, Report Series 11, No. 1, *Cocaine*, January, 1972, p. 3; *STASH Fact Sheet on Cocaine*, Grassroots (February, 1972 Supplement), p. 1.

9. Terence Clark, "Cocaine," Texas Medicine, Vol. 69, 1973, p. 74; Sigmund Freud, "Uber Coca" *Central Journal for Therapy*, Vienna, July, 1884; Gerald T. McLaughlin, "Cocaine: The History and Regulation of a Dangerous Drug," *58 Cornell Law Review*, March, 1973, p. 544; and Mortimer, op. cit., p. 16.

10. Henry Brill, "Recurrent Patterns in the History of Drugs," in *Drugs and Youth, Proceedings of the Rutgers Symposium on Drug Abuse* (Springfield: Charles C. Thomas, 1969), p. 11; The Encyclopedia Americana, "Cocaine," (New York: Americana Corporation, 1938); T. E. Keys, *The History of Surgical Anesthesia* (New York: Dover Publishers, 1963), pp. 38-44; Norman Taylor, op. cit., p. 14; J. H. Woods and D. A. Downs, op. cit., p. 117.

11. J. H. Woods and D. A. Downs, op. cit., p. 117.

12. Sigmund Freud, op. cit.

13. Ibid.

14. Ibid.

15. Ibid.

16. Ibid.

17. Ibid.

18. Ibid.

19. Edward Brecher, *Licit & Illicit Drugs* (Boston: Little, Brown and Company, 1972), p. 279.

20. Ernest Jones, *The Life and Work of Sigmund Freud, Volume I* (New York: Basic Books, 1961), p. 52.

21. Ibid.

22. Ibid., p. 53.

23. Ibid., p. 57.

24. Ibid., p. 53.

25. Freud, op. cit.

26. Jones, op. cit., p. 54.

27. Freud, op. cit.

28. Jones, op. cit., p. 54.

29. Quoted in "The Growing Menace of the Use of Cocaine," *The New York Times,* August 2, 1908.

30. Jones, op. cit., p. 55.

31. Ibid., p. 57.

32. The term "psychopharmacology" was apparently coined by the pharmacologist David Macht in 1920.

33. Compare, for example, the relevant data offered in L. S. Goodman and A. Gilman, *The Pharmacological Basis of Therapeutics* (4th ed.; New York: The Macmillan Co., 1970).

34. Sigmund Freud, op. cit.

35. Freud, op. cit., *Addenda.*

36. Freud, op. cit.

37. See Chapter III.

38. The earliest reference to such use I have found is in Aleister Crowley's 1922 novel, *Diary of a Drug Fiend* (New York: Samuel Weiser, Inc., 1973).

39. Jones, op. cit., p. 63.

40. Ibid., p. 62.

41. Ibid.

42. Freud, op. cit.

43. Ibid.

44. See Chapter VIII.

45. Brecher, op. cit., p. 275.

46. In *Uber Coca,* Freud asserts cocaine has no such cumulative effect.

47. See Chapter VIII.

48. Emil Erlenmeyer, cited in Jones, op. cit., p. 64.

49. Sigmund Freud, "Craving For and Fear of Cocaine," *Wiener medizinische Wochenschrift,* July 9, 1887; and in Freud, *The Cocaine Papers* (Vienna: Dunguin Press, 1963).

50. Sigmund Freud, *The Interpretation of Dreams* in *The Basic Writings of Sigmund Freud* (New York: The Modern Library, 1938), p. 199.

51. In *The Gourmet Cokebook* (White Mountain Press, Inc., 1972), p. 15.

52. And the operations were on the palate and jaw. See Brecher, op. cit., pp. 214-215.

53. A Hrdlicka, "Trephination Among Prehistoric People," Ciba Symposia, Vol. I, No. 6, 1939; and *History of Medicine in Pictures*, Vol. 4 (Parke, Davis & Co., 1960).

54. J. H. Woods and D. A. Downs, op. cit., p. 118.
55. H. K. Becker, op. cit., p. 320.
56. Ibid., p. 323.
57. Ibid.
58. J. H. Woods and D. A. Downs, op. cit., p. 117.
59. Freud, op. cit., *Uber Coca.*
60. Ibid.
61. H. K. Becker, op. cit., p. 234.
62. Ibid.
63. Ibid.
64. Freud, op. cit.
65. Ibid.
66. Freud, op. cit., *Addenda.*
67. Sigmund Freud, "Contribution to the Knowledge of the Effect of Cocaine," *The Cocaine Papers* (Vienna: Dunguin Press, 1963).
68. Edward Brecher, op. cit., p. 33.
69. Charles Perry, "The Star-Spangled Powder, or Through History with Coke Spoon and Nasal Spray," *Rolling Stone,* Issue No. 115, August 17, 1972.
70. Wilder Penfield, "Halsted of Johns Hopkins, The Man and His Problem as Described in the Secret Records of William Osler," *JAMA,* 210 (December 22, 1969), p. 2215.
71. Ibid.
72. Edward Brecher, op. cit., pp. 33-35.

Chapter III

1. G. Archie Stockwell, "Erythroxylon Coca," *Boston Med. Surg. J. 96:* 402, 1887, cited in David Musto, *The American Disease, Origins of Narcotic Control* (New Haven: Yale University Press, 1973).
2. W. A. Hammond, "Remarks on Cocaine and the So-Called Cocaine Habit," *J. Nerv. & Ment. Dis.,* 13:754, 1886.
3. Sir Robert Christison, "Observations on the effect of Cuca, or coca, etc.," *British Medical Journal,* 1870. (Cited in Freud, "Uber Coca.")
4. Emil Erlenmeyer, who criticized Freud in the *Centralblatt for Newenheilkunde,* a professional journal he edited. (Cited in Ernest Jones, *The Life and Work*

of *Sigmund Freud, Volume I.* New York: Basic Books, 1961, p. 63.)

5. Sir Arthur Conan Doyle, *A Scandal in Bohemia.*

6. Myron G. Schultz, "The 'Strange Case' of Robert Louis Stevenson," *Journal of the American Medical Association,* April 5, 1971, Vol. 216, p. 91.

7. W. G. Mortimer, *Peru History of Coca, "The Divine Plant" of the Incas* (New York: J. H. Vail and Company, 1901), p. 177. Hereinafter cited as *Mortimer.*

8. Ibid., p. 180.

9. Ibid., p. 179.

10. Ibid., p. 180.

11. W. C. Burke & D. J. Hall, "Blessing From Hell, Koller and Cocaine," in Chapter IV of M. Silverman, *The War Against Disease,* 1942.

12. H. K. Becker, "Carl Koller and Cocaine," *The Psychoanalytic Quarterly,* Vol. 32, No. 3, 1963, p. 322.

13. *Mortimer,* p. 180.

14. Ibid.

15. Becker, op. cit., says 1863. As for the 1865 possibility, due to a mishap which occurred during the moving of household goods, the citation has been lost and I have been unable to recover it.

16. Norman Taylor, *Plant Drugs That Changed the World* (New York: Dodd, Mead & Company, 1965), p. 12.

17. Angelo Mariani, *Coca and Its Therapeutic Application,* New York, 1896.

18. Taylor, op. cit., p. 12 and Becker, op. cit., p. 322.

19. *Mortimer,* p. 178.

20. Ibid., p. 179.

21. Ibid., p. 180.

22. Becker, op. cit., p. 322.

23. Edward Brecher, *Licit & Illicit Drugs* (Boston: Little, Brown and Company, 1972), p. 31.

24. For an illuminating discussion of the general situation with respect to the practices of parent and proprietary medicine manufacturers see J. H. Young, *The Toadstool Millionaires* (Princeton: Princeton University Press, Princeton Paperback Ed. 1972).

25. *Mortimer,* p. 178.

26. E. J. Kahn, *The Big Drink: The Story of Coca-Cola* (New York: Random House, 1960).

27. Kahn, op. cit., and Musto, op. cit., Chapter I and the notes thereto.

28. For the extent of the industry see J. H. Young, op. cit.

29. Due to a mishap which occurred during the moving of household goods, the primary source has been lost. But *The Gourmet Cokebook* (White Mountain Press, Inc., 1972) carries the reproduction of what it says is an advertisement for Metcalf's Coca Wine from a turn-of-the-century medical journal which contains the quoted words.

30. *Nostrums and Quackery*, Articles on the Nostrum Evil and Quackery Reprinted, with Additions and Modifications, from the *Journal of the American Medical Association* (Chicago: American Medical Association, 1912), 2nd Ed., p. 429.

31. Ibid.

32. Ibid.

33. Ibid.

34. Ibid.

35. Ibid., p. 551.

36. Ibid., p. 535.

37. Ibid., p. 537.

38. Steward H. Hobrook, *The Golden Age of Quackery* (New York: The Macmillan Co., 1959), p. 52.

39. *Nostrums and Quackery,* op. cit., pp. 530-537, 543, 546, 553, 563.

40. Ibid., p. 530.

41. For example, when I was a child in Belleville, Ontario, a town some 100 miles east of Toronto, "dope" was the term for Coca-Cola in 1939.

42. J. H. Young, op. cit., p. 109.

43. "Nations Uniting to Stamp Out the Use of Opium and Many Other Drugs," *The New York Times,* July 25, 1909.

44. Estimate supplied by an agent of the Drug Enforcement Agency, March, 1974.

45. "Report of Committee on the Acquirement of Drug Habits," *75 American Journal of Pharmacy,* 1903, p. 486.

46. "The Growing Menace of the Use of Cocaine," *The New York Times*, August 2, 1908.
47. J. H. Young, op. cit., pp. 219-222.
48. See Chapter IV.
49. *The New York Times*, op. cit., July 25, 1909 and "More Than 1,000,000 Drug Users in U.S.," *The New York Times*, June 13, 1919.
50. J. H. Young, op. cit., p. 248.
51. Ibid., p. 243.
52. David E. Smith and Donald R. Wesson, "Legitimate and illegitimate distribution of amphetamines and barbiturates," in *Uppers and Downers* (Englewood Cliffs, N. H.: Prentice-Hall, Inc., 1973), pp. 108-117.
53. *The New York Times*, May 3, 1974, p. 49.
54. Ibid.
55. David Musto, *The American Disease, Origins of Narcotic Control* (New Haven: Yale University Press, 1973), p. 7.

Chapter IV

1. David Musto, "A Study in Cocaine, Sherlock Holmes and Sigmund Freud," *Journal of the American Medical Association*, April 1, 1968, Vol. 204, No. 1, p. 126.
2. See Chapter VIII for the relative innocuousness of cocaine and various reports issued by the National Institute on Alcohol Abuse and Alcoholism, National Institute of Mental Health concerning the serious repercussions of alcohol use in America. (Estimates of alcoholism—i.e., *addiction* to alcohol—range from 5,000,000 to 10,000,000.)
3. *Marihuana, A Signal of Misunderstanding*, the Official Report of the National Commission on Marihuana and Drug Abuse, Part V.
4. Oregon.
5. See the relevant sections in Edward Brecher, *Licit & Illicit Drugs* (Boston: Little, Brown and Company, 1972).
6. Charles B. Towns, "The Peril of the Drug Habit," *Century Magazine*, 84 (1912), p. 586.

7. Louis Lewin, *Phantastica: Narcotic and Stimulating Drugs: Their Use and Abuse*, 1924, p. 80.

8. "Cocaine Used Most by Drug Addicts," *The New York Times*, April 15, 1926.

9. "The Growing Menace of the Use of Cocaine," *The New York Times*, August 2, 1908.

10. Robert S. deRopp, *Drugs and the Mind* (New York: Grove Press, Inc., 1961), p. 248.

11. Emil Erlenmeyer, cited in Ernest Jones, *The Life and Work of Sigmund Freud, Volume I* (New York: Basic Books, 1961), p. 63.

12. Jones, op. cit., p. 63.

13. Ibid., p. 64.

14. Ibid.

15. Ibid.

16. J. B. Mattison, "Cocaine Poisoning," *Medical and Surgical Reporter*, 65, 1891, pp. 645-650.

17. J. H. Woods and D. A. Downs, "The Psychopharmacology of Cocaine," in *Drug use in America: problem in perspective, the Technical Papers of the Second Report of the National Commission on Marijuana and Drug Abuse* (Washington, D.C.: U. S. Government Printing Office, March, 1973), p. 124.

18. See Chapter VIII.

19. See note 2.

20. Edward Marshall, "Uncle Sam Is the Worst Drug Fiend in the World," *The New York Times*, March 12, 1911.

21. Charles Terry and Mildred Pellens, *The Opium Problem* (New York: Committee on Drug Addictions, Bureau of Social Hygiene, Inc., 1928), p. 28.

22. Edward Marshall, op. cit.

23. Ibid.

24. J. H. Young, *The Toadstool Millionaires* (Princeton: Princeton University Press, Princeton Paperback Editions, 1972), pp. 158-159.

25. Ibid., p. 158.

26. Ibid., p. 209.

27. Ibid.

28. Ibid., p. 207.

29. Ibid.

30. Ibid.

31. Ibid.

32. Ibid., p. 234.
33. Ibid.
34. Ibid., p. 224.
35. "The Growing Menace of the Use of Cocaine," op. cit.
36. Ibid.
37. Lucius P. Brown, "Enforcement of the Tennessee Anti-Narcotics Law," *American Journal of Public Health* Vol. 5 (April, 1915), p. 324.
38. "The Cocaine Habit Among Negroes," *The British Medical Journal,* Nov. 29, 1902, p. 1729.
39. Edward Huntington Williams, "Negro Cocaine 'Fiends' Are a New Southern Menace," *The New York Times,* February 8, 1914.
40. W. Scheppegrell, "The Abuse and Dangers of Cocaine," *Medical News,* Vol. 73, 1898, pp. 417-422.
41. Editorial, *Journal of the American Medical Association,* Vol. 34, June, 1900, p. 1637. See also *JAMA,* Vol. 36, February, 1901, p. 330.
42. "The Cocaine Habit Among Negroes," op. cit.
43. David Musto, *The American Disease, Origins of Narcotic Control* (New Haven: Yale University Press, 1973), p. 7.
44. Ibid.
45. *The New York Tribune,* June 21, 1903.
46. *Report of the President's Homes Commission,* Senate Document No. 644, 60th Congress, 2nd Session (Washington, D. C.: Government Printing Office, January 8, 1909), pp. 254-255.
47. David Musto, op. cit., note 15, p. 254.
48. David Musto, op. cit.
49. *Literary Digest,* March 28, 1914, p. 687.
50. David Musto, op. cit.
51. Edward Huntington Williams, op. cit.
52. Ibid.
53. Heard on either WCBS or WOR, New York, on June 21 or 22, 1974.
54. E. M. Green, "Psychoses Among Negroes: A Comparative Study," *Journal of Nervous and Mental Disorders,* Vol. 41, 1914, pp. 697-708.
55. David Musto, op. cit., pp. 14-21.
56. Edward Huntington Williams, op. cit.

57. "The Growing Menace of the Use of Cocaine," op. cit.

58. Ibid.

59. "Cocaine Used Most by Drug Addicts," op. cit.

60. "Nations Uniting to Stamp Out the Use of Opium and Many Other Drugs," *The New York Times,* July 25, 1909.

61. Ibid.

62. "The Growing Menace of the Use of Cocaine," op. cit.

63. See E. C. Sandmeyer, *The Anti-Chinese Movement in California* (Urbana: University of Illinois Press, 1939).

64. See Ashley, *Heroin, The Myths and the Facts* (New York: St. Martin's Press, 1972), pp. 114-115.

65. *U. S. Treasury Department, State Laws Relating to the Control of Narcotic Drugs and the Treatment of Drug Addiction,* 1931, part III.

66. Ibid.

67. Ibid.

68. Ibid.

69. Ibid.

70. Gerald T. McLaughlin, "Cocaine: The History and Regulation of a Dangerous Drug," *Cornell Law Review,* Vol. 58, March, 1973, p. 562.

71. Ibid.

72. Ibid., p. 563.

73. Ibid., pp. 570-571.

74. Ibid., p. 568.

75. R. Ashley, June 24, 1974.

76. Pendleton King, *Cocaine (A Play in One Act).*

77. Judge Garrity, *Memorandum and Order Denying Motions to Reduce,* February 26, 1974 in United States of America v. Foss and Coveney, Criminal No. 73-24-G, United States District Court, District of Massachusetts.

Chapter V

1. Alfred R. Lindesmith, *The Addict and the Law* (New York: Vintage Books, 1965), p. 99.

2. "Seize 'Coke King' and $50,000 Drugs," *The New York Times,* September 6, 1924, p. 12.

3. "Dr. Simon and a Detective Arrest the 'Cocaine King' After a Long Hunt," *The New York Times,* April 2, 1921, p. 4.

4. Wolcott Gibbs, *More in Sorrow* (New York: Henry Holt and Company, 1958), pp. 140-141.

5. Quoted in David Musto, "A Study in Cocaine, Sherlock Holmes and Sigmund Freud," *Journal of the American Medical Association,* April 1, 1968, Vol. 204, No. 1, p. 126.

6. *Proceedings of the American Pharmaceutical Association 51,* 1903, p. 477.

7. Ibid.

8. Ibid.

9. "Finds Drug Evil Pervades the City," *The New York Times,* December 5, 1916.

10. *Traffic in Narcotic Drugs*—Report of Special Committee of Investigation appointed March 25, 1918, by the Secretary of the Treasury, (Washington, 1919).

11. Charles Terry and Mildred Pellans, *The Opium Problem* (New York Committee on Drug Addictions, Bureau of Social Hygiene Inc., 1928), p. 32.

12. Commission on Public Health, New York Academy of Medicine, *39 Report on Drug Addiction—II,* (1963), p. 432.

13. Joseph McIver and George E. Price, "Drug Addiction, Analysis of 147 Cases at the Philadelphia General Hospital," *Journal of the American Medical Association,* February 12, 1916, p. 477.

14. Edward Brecher, *Licit & Illicit Drugs* (Boston: Little, Brown and Company, 1972), p. 38.

15. See Chapter VIII.

16. *The New York Times,* December 6, 1916.

17. "Dr. Copeland Reports Great Increase in Sale of Habit-Forming Drugs Here," *The New York Times,* March 23, 1919.

18. "The Growing Menace of the Use of Cocaine," *The New York Times,* August 2, 1908.

19. "Police Drive Raises Price of Cocaine," *The New York Times,* February 1, 1930, p. 10.

20. Lee Israel, *Miss Tallulah Bankhead* (New York: G. P. Putnam's Sons, 1973), p. 75.

21. Ibid., p. 74.

22. Personal communication, March, 1974.

23. See Richard Woodley, *Dealer, Portrait of a Cocaine Merchant* (New York: Warner Paperback Library, 1972).

24. Quoted in David Musto, *The American Disease* (New Haven: Yale University Press, 1973), p. 15.

25. *The New York Times,* January 22, 1914.

26. "Cocaine Used Most by Drug Addicts," *The New York Times,* April 25, 1926.

27. Before the Harrison Act, when the opiates were very cheap, the typical addict was relatively affluent. After Harrison, as black market conditions drove prices up, the typical addict more and more was drawn from the poorer classes. See Richard Ashley, *Heroin, The Myths and the Facts* (New York: St. Martin's Press, 1972), pp. 49-56.

28. "Happy Days in Hollywood," *Vanity Fair,* May, 1922, p. 73.

29. See Benjamin B. Hampton, *A History of the Movies* (New York: Covici-Friede, 1931), pp. 284-297.

30. Ibid.

31. Ibid.

32. "Wally Reid Better; Wife Talks of Case," *The New York Times,* December 19, 1922.

33. Gene Fowler, *Father Goose, The Story of Mack Sennett* (New York: Covici-Friede, 1934), p. 319.

34. "Wally Reid Better; Wife Talks of Case," op. cit.

35. "The Cocaine Traffic in India," *The New York Times Current History,* Vol. 16, September, 1922, p. 949.

36. I. C. Chopra and R. N. Chopra, "The Cocaine Problem in India," United Nations *Bulletin on Narcotics,* April-June, 1958, p. 15.

37. Col. Ahmed A. El Hadka, "Forty Years of the Campaign Against Narcotic Drugs in the United Arab Republic," United Nations *Bulletin on Narcotics.*

38. "Spread of Drug Habit Alarms Berlin Police," *The New York Times,* August 16, 1925.

39. Ibid.

40. Louis Lewin, *Phantastica: Narcotic and Stimulating Drugs: Their Use and Abuse*, 1924, p. 80.

41. "Huge Narcotic Ring Smashed in Berlin," *The New York Times*, September 14, 1926.

42. "Ex-German Officers Held in Big Drug Plot," *The New York Times*, February 21, 1927.

43. "Soldiers Smuggle Cocaine to French," *The New York Times*, June 24, 1921.

44. Ibid.

45. "The Nightmare of Cocaine" (By a former "Snow-Bird"), *The North American Review*, Vol. 227, April, 1929, p. 419.

46. Marcel Proust, *The Captive* (New York: The Modern Library, 1929), p. 309.

47. Marcel Proust, *The Past Recaptured* (New York: Modern Library, 1932), p. 130.

48. Ibid., p. 283.

49. "Fight Drug Evil in 2 Hemispheres," *The New York Times*, November 5, 1916.

50. Ibid.

51. Aleister Crowley, *The Diary of a Drug Fiend*, (New York: Samuel Weiser Inc., 1973, reprint of 1922 ed.), p. 289.

52. Nathan Mutch, "Cocaine," *Guy's Hospital Gazette*, Vol. 46, 1932, p. 425.

53. Aleister Crowley, op. cit., p. 144.

54. Ibid., p. 50.

55. Ibid., p. 26.

56. Ibid., p. 44.

57. Ibid., p. 287.

58. Ibid., p. 48.

59. Ibid., p. 53.

60. Ibid., p. 244.

61. Ibid., p. 289.

Chapter VI

1. Hayes and Bower, "Marihuana," *Journal of Criminal Law and Criminology*, Vol. 23, 1932, p. 1088. Quoted in Bonnie and Whitebread, "The Forbidden Fruit and the Tree of Knowledge: An Inquiry into

the Legal History of the American Marihuana Prohibition," *56 Virginia Law Review,* October, 1970.

2. Ibid., emphasis added.

3. *Hearing on H.R. 6385 Before the House Committee on Ways and Means,* 75th Congress, 1st Session, 1937, p. 32. Quoted in Bonnie and Whitebread, "The Forbidden Fruit and the Tree of Knowledge: An Inquiry into the Legal History of the American Marihuana Prohibition," *56 Virginia Law Review,* October, 1970.

4. Recorded in Memphis, Tennessee, 1930. (Victor v. 38620).

5. Personal communication, January, 1974.

6. *The Gourmet Cokebook* (White Mountain Press, Inc., 1972), p. 25.

7. Joachim C. Fest, *Hitler* (New York: Harcourt Brace Jovanovich, Inc., 1974), p. 740.

8. Ibid., pp. 667-674.

9. Ibid., p. 672.

10. Ibid., p. 673.

11. Edward Brecher, *Licit & Illicit Drugs* (Boston: Little, Brown and Company, 1972), p. 278.

12. *Physician's Desk Reference to Pharmaceutical Specialties and Biologicals* (26th Ed.; Oradell, New Jersey: Medical Economics, 1972) and Sidney Cohen, "Control of Drug Abuse," *34 Federal Probation,* March, 1970.

13. Iago Galdston, "Pep Teasers," *Hygeia,* Vol. 18, October, 1940, pp. 878-880. (Cited in Brecher, op. cit., p. 280).

14. Edward Brecher, op. cit., p. 281.

15. Ibid., p. 282.

16. *Time,* April 11, 1949, p. 44.

17. United Nations, *Bulletin on Narcotics,* July-September, 1962, p. 11.

18. Ibid.

19. United Nations, *Bulletin on Narcotics,* October-December, 1964, p. 44.

20. *The New York Times,* December 18, 1964.

21. "World Drug Traffic and Its Impact on U. S. Security," *Hearings Before the Subcommittee of the Committee on the Judiciary to Investigate the Administration of the Internal Security Act and Other*

Internal Security Laws, U. S. Senate, 92nd Congress,
2nd Session, September 18, 1972, (Washington,
D. C.: U. S. Government Printing Office, 1972),
p. 295.

22. Ibid.
23. Ibid.
24. "Cocaine is Re-Emerging as a Major Problem, While
    Marijuana Remains Popular," *The New York Times,*
    November 15, 1971.
25. Ibid.
26. J. T. Gossett, J. M. Lewis, and V. A. Phillips, "Ex-
    tent and Prevalence of Illicit Drug Use as Reported
    by 56,745 Students," *Journal of the American Medi-
    cal Association,* Vol. 216, No. 9, May 31, 1971,
    p. 1465.
27. Dorothy F. Berg, "Dangerous Drugs in the United
    States," *International Journal of the Addictions,* Vol.
    5 (4), 1970, p. 809.
28. "An Assessment of Drug Use in the General Popula-
    tions," *Special Report No. 1, Drug Use in New York
    State* (New York State Narcotic Addiction Control
    Commission), May 1971, pp. 136-142.
29. Due to a mishap which occurred during the moving
    of household goods, the citation was lost.
30. Mary Hager, "One in 10 addicts using Cocaine: U. S.
    survey," *The Journal* (Addiction Research Founda-
    tion), 2 (4), April 1, 1973.
31. C.F. Karl Marx, *Capital* (1867), Vol. I.
32. In the *Journal of the American Medical Association,*
    Vol. 204, No. 1, April 1, 1968.
33. According to *Variety, Easy Rider* grossed $16,000,-
    000 in America while *Lawrence of Arabia* grossed
    $15,000,000 and *A Man for All Seasons* $12,750,000.
34. Among them: Spiro Agnew and all the F.C.C. com-
    missioners except Nicholas Johnson.
35. *Newsweek,* September 27, 1971.
36. *Rolling Stone,* issue No. 81, April 29, 1971.
37. Ibid.
38. Richard Woodley, *Dealer, Portrait of a Cocaine Mer-
    chant* (New York: Warner Paperback Library,
    1972).
39. "Smuggling: The Medicine Men," *Newsweek,* June
    12, 1972.

40. Charles Perry, "The Star-Spangled Powder, or, Through History with Coke Spoon and Nasal Spray," *Rolling Stone*, Issue No. 115, August 17, 1972.

41. *The Gourmet Cokebook* (White Mountain Press, Inc., 1972).

42. Bruce Jay Friedman, *About Harry Towns* (New York: Alfred A. Knopf, 1974), p. 77.

43. Ibid.

44. Thomas Plate, "Coke: The Big New Easy-Entry Business," *New York,* Vol. 6, No. 45, November 5, 1973.

45. Personal communication from a DEA agent, February, 1974.

46. Marc Olden, *Cocaine* (New York: Lancer Books, 1973), p. 66.

47. Ibid., p. 81.

48. Ibid., p. 105.

49. Ibid., p. 170.

50. *The World Narcotics Problem: The Latin American Perspective,* Report of Special Study Mission to Latin America and the Federal Republic of Germany, pursuant to H. Res. 267, 93rd Congress, 1st Session (Washington: U. S. Government Printing Office, 1973), p. 1.

Chapter VII

1. See Appendix II.

2. M. A. Farber, "Drug Traffic Thriving Despite New Stiff Law," *The New York Times,* October 8, 1973.

3. M. A. Farber, "Narcotic Arrests Drop 75% in City," *The New York Times,* October 1, 1973.

4. For the counter-productive aspects of severe penalties see *Deterrent Effects of Criminal Sanctions,* Progress Report of the Assembly Committee on Criminal Procedure (Assembly of the State of California, May, 1968; Jerome Skolnick, "Coercion to Virtue: The Enforcement of Morals," *41 Southern California Law Review,* 588 (1968); Bonnie & Whitebread, "The Forbidden Fruit and the Tree of Knowledge: An Inquiry into the Legal History of

American Marihuana Prohibition," *56 Virginia Law Review* (October, 1970), pp. 1133-1140.

5. From an interview, September, 1973.
6. Personal communication, Drug Enforcement Administration agent, February, 1974.
7. Ibid.
8. J. H. Woods and D. A. Downs, "The Psychopharmacology of Cocaine," *Drug Use in America: Problem in Perspective, the Technical Papers of the Second Report of the National Commission on Marihuana and Drug Abuse,* Vol. I, March, 1973, p. 130.
9. Richard Ashley, *Heroin, The Myths and the Facts* (New York: St. Martin's Press, 1972), pp. 29-30, 160.
10. See Chapter I and Chapter VIII.

Chapter VIII

1. James H. Woods and David A. Downs, "The Psychopharmacology of Cocaine," *Drug Use in America: Problem in Perspective, the Technical Papers of the Second Report of the National Commission on Marihuana and Drug Abuse,* Vol. I, March, 1973, pp. 116-139.
2. L. A. Woods *et al.,* "Distribution and Metabolism of Cocaine in the Dog and the Rabbit," *Journal of Pharmacology and Experimental Therapeutics,* Vol. 101, 1951, pp. 200-204.
3. Ibid.
4. Ibid.
5. D. Campbell and S. Adriani, "Absorption of Local Anesthetics," *Journal of the American Medical Association,* Vol. 168, 1958, pp. 873-877.
6. L. A. Woods *et al.,* op. cit.
7. R. T. Williams, *Detoxication Mechanisms* (New York: John Wiley & Son Inc.), 1959), p. 557.
8. Woods and Downs, op. cit., pp. 120-121.
9. Louis S. Goodman and Alfred Gilman, eds., *The Pharmacological Basis of Therapeutics* (4th ed.; New York: The Macmillan Co., 1970), p. 381.
10. Woods and Downs, op. cit., pp. 128-129.
11. Ibid., p. 122.

12. Goodman and Gilman, op. cit., p. 380.
13. E.g. Goodman and Gilman.
14. Reported in A. R. McIntyre, "Renal Excretion of Cocaine in a Case of Acute Cocaine Poisoning," *Journal of Pharmacology and Experimental Therapeutics*, Vol. 57, 1936, p. 133.
15. Goodman and Gilman, op. cit., p. 380.
16. Sigmund Freud, "Contribution to the Knowledge of the Effect of Cocaine," *The Cocaine Papers* (Vienna: Dunguin Press, 1963).
17. Goodman and Gilman, op. cit.
18. E.g. Sigmund Freud, W. G. Mortimer, Richard Ashley.
19. Sigmund Freud, "Uber Coca," op. cit.
20. The bulk (63) of the interviews were done between October, 1972 and November, 1973, the remainder took place between December, 1973 and May of 1974. Only a very few of the subjects were seen less than twice and 21 were seen on three or more occasions. In 15 cases, the cocaine used had been submitted to a testing laboratory to ascertain its purity; in all other cases purity was tested by several of the methods outlined in Chapter VII. Unfortunately, most of the raw data was lost during the moving of household goods—otherwise a sizable appendix would have been included. Fortunately I had abstracted most of the relevant data prior to the loss. All of the samples, with the exception of one man, were current users of marijuana; 75 were current users of alcohol; and 72 had used or still used the more potent psychedelics. Twenty-six of the sample were female, 55 were male, 37 were between the ages of 30 and 45, 40 between 21 and 29, 3 between 18 and 20, and 1 was 16. Fifteen of the sample were drug dealers, 22 were musicians, and the remainder included lawyers, doctors, teachers, garment salesman, dress designers, models, advertising copywriters, art directors, account executives, photographers, hairdressers, stock brokers, journalists, editors, authors, and housewives. None of the samples was a current user of heroin, although 3 had used it in the past. The absence of heroin users from the sample was deliberate, since it has been my experi-

ence that heroin users do not use cocaine for its own sake but rather for the way it affects the heroin experience.

21. Male, 28 years of age, interviewed on May 14, 1974.

22. In Volume 3, p. 552.

23. Torald Sollmann, *A Manual of Pharmacology* (6th ed.; Philadelphia: W. B. Saunders Company, 1942), p. 322.

24. *British Pharmaceutical Codex* (London: The Pharmaceutical Press, 1963), p. 197.

25. Goodman and Gilman, op. cit., p. 381.

26. *National Clearinghouse for Drug Abuse Information*, Report Series II, No. 1, *Cocaine*, January, 1972, pp. 7-8.

27. E.g. the World Health Organization (WHO) definition previously cited. For an interesting discussion of WHO's shifting-the-grounds tactics in this respect see J. Zacune, "What's in a name?" *Drugs and Society*, Vol. I, No. 4, January, 1972.

28. Edward Brecher, *Licit & Illicit Drugs* (Boston: Little, Brown and Company), p. 276.

29. Edward Brecher, paragraph 9 of Affidavit attached to *Defendant's Joint Memorandum in Support of Their Motions for Correction or Reduction of Sentence* (United States of America v. Foss and Coveney, U. S. District Court, District of Massachusetts: Criminal No. 73-24-G), 1974.

30. Dr. Norman Zinberg, paragraph 3 of Affidavit, attached to *Joint Memorandum* cited above.

31. James V. DeLong, "The Drugs and Their Effects," in *Dealing With Drug Abuse, A Report to the Ford Foundation* (New York: Praeger Publishers, 1972), p. 105.

32. Personal communications.

33. Sigmund Freud, "Craving For and Fear of Cocaine," op. cit.

34. J. B. Mattison, "Cocaine Poisoning," *Medical and Surgical Reporter*, Vol. 65, 1891, pp. 645-650.

35. E. Mayer, "The Toxic Effects Following the Use of Local Anesthetics," *Journal of the American Medical Association*, Vol. 82, 1924, pp. 876-885.

36. Woods and Downs, op. cit., p. 124.

37. Ibid.

38. Goodman and Gilman, op. cit., p. 381.
39. Woods and Downs, op. cit.
40. Ibid.
41. Ibid., p. 125.
42. Andrew T. Weil, "Altered States of Consciousness," in *Dealing With Drug Abuse, A Report to the Ford Foundation* (New York: Praeger Publishers, 1972), p. 330.
43. Senator Edward Kennedy, Chairman of the Health Subcommittee of the Senate Labor and Public Welfare Committee, quoted in *The New York Times,* May 21, 1974.

Index

Acosta, Joseph de, 17

Adams, Samuel Hopkins, 65, 79

Addiction. See Drug addiction

Alcohol, 14, 70, 75, 132; addiction to, 25, 76, 155; prohibition on, 73, 81, 131, 203–204

Alkaloids: discovery of, 32, 33; properties of, 31–32

American Medical Association (AMA), 78, 79; Journal of, 79, 82, 134, 135

American Pharmaceutical Association, 78, 107; Committee on the Acquirement of the Drug Habit of, 87

Amphetamines, 34, 68, 71, 107, 125, 126, 133, 155, 179

Anesthetics, 40, 41–46

Anslinger, Harry, 120, 127

Anticocaine laws, 63, 66, 116–117, 118. See also Cocaine; Drug laws

Antidrug laws. See Drug laws

Antidrug literature, 100

Anything Goes, 110

Arbuckle, Fatty, 111

Aschenbrandt, Theodor, 34, 35

Ashley, Richard, 131

Aspirin, 66

Atropine, 31, 32

Axton, Hoyt, 135

AZ-MA-SYDE, 62–63

Bankhead, Tallulah, 105

Barbiturates, 67, 133

Barkham, Henry, 16

Baudelaire, C. P., 133

Bentley, W. H., 34

Bernays, Martha, 35

Bishop, Ernest, 101, 102

248

Brecher, Edward, 25, 131, 177

British Medical Journal, 82

Brown, Lucius P., 80

Bureau of Narcotics and Dangerous Drugs, 129, 140, 179

Burroughs, William, 116

Caffeine, 31, 32

Campbell, Jackson R., 108

Cash, Johnny, 134

Chaplin, Charlie, 109, 110

Christison, Robert, 50

Chronica del Peru, 16

Cieza de Leon, Pedro, 16

Cinchona, 17

Coca:
amount of cocaine in, 27–28, 31; ban on importing, 91–92; beliefs about, 19–20, 23–25; effects of, 18, 22–25, 44, 167–168; origins of, 15, 19, 74; production of, 25–26; prohibition on use of, 21–22; use, and illiteracy, 23; use, and malnutrition, 24; varieties of, 27; vitamins in, 27; western discovery of, 16–18, 32–33. *See also* Cocaine

Coca-Bola, 62

Coca-Cola, 59–60, 63, 64, 83

Cocaine:
addiction, 46–47, 77, 155–156, 167, 173, 174–176; amount of, extracted from coca, 27–28, 31; appearance of, 158–159; as treatment for morphine addiction, 34, 36, 39, 51–52, 58, 74, 76; attitudes toward, 122–124; availability of, 59; burning of, 160–161; classed as a narcotic, 91, 92, 93, 94, 95–96; cuts of, 159–162; dealing, 147–154; discovery of, 32–33; duties on, 64; effects of, 22, 28–29, 35, 38–39, 40, 47, 50, 54, 59, 60, 67, 71, 87–88, 100–101, 117–118, 157, 162, 164–185; estimating number of users of, 129–130, 142; Freud's research on, 36–37, 40–41, 44–45, 71, 169; Freud's use of, 35–38, 39–41, 48; government control of, 127, 140–141; historical outline of, 217–221; legislation against, 89–94; markets, 145, 146, 147, 152–155, 158; measuring, 226–227; medical uses of, 18, 34, 38–39, 40–47, 56, 180; misconceptions about, 23, 94–96, 102, 140–141, 175–176, 186–189; 19th century marketing of, 54–58; in patent medicines, 59–64; 'pharmaceutical', 159, 160; physiological effects of, 165–169; poisoning, 39; popularizing of, 50–58, 69, 119, 126–127, 129–130, 142; prices, 65, 104–105, 108, 122, 143–144, 155–158; production of, 205–208, psychoactive effects of, 169–177, 183; purity of, 158–162, 213–

214; quality of, 153–154; rate of use of, 64–66; refining of, 27, 159, 160–161; research, 33–34, 36–38, 40, 44–45, 71, 178–179, 181–183; research (Freud's), 36–38, 40–41, 44–45, 71, 169; scarcity of, 156; seizures of, in recent years, 128; sensationalism about, 111–112, 120, 135–137, 139; snorting, 161–162; sources of, 147; storage of, 219–220; suppression of, 15, 65–66, 89–93; taste of, 160; toxic and adverse reactions to, 180–182, 211–212; traffic abroad, 112–114, 116–117, 125; transformation of, into a dangerous drug, 70–89, 93; use, decline in, 125–126; use, estimating, 129–130, 142; use, rate of, 64–66; use, social patterns of, 97–98, 102–104, 107–118, 119–125, 132–139; use, by blacks, 73, 81–89, 106–107; use, by criminals, 89, 107–108; use, by whites, 72–73, 87–88, 107; used as a local anesthetic, 40, 41–46, 56, 167; used as a stimulant, 41, 58; uses, medical, 18, 34, 38–39, 40–46, 56, 180–181; ways of taking, 165–166, 171, 179; weighing, 158

Cocaine, 94

Cocaine Fiends, The, 123, 124

Cocaine Papers, 142

Coca leaves, 15, 32
Coca shrub, 25
Coffee, 14, 73
Collier's magazine, 79
Collins, Cornelius F., 104
Comprehensive Drug Abuse Prevention and Control Act of 1970, 92, 187
Consumers Union Report, on *Licit & Illicit Drugs*, 24
Copeland, Royal S., 104
Corning, J. Leonard, 36, 56
Craving For and Fear of Cocaine, 37, 41
Crowley, Aleister, 117, 137
Cubans, in the drug market, 152–153

Dain Curse, The, 52
Damiana, 63
De Jussieu, A. L., 33
Detroit Therapeutic Gazette, 34, 35
Downs, David A., 165
Doyle, Arthur Conan, 51, 52, 53, 54, 94, 137
Dr. Tucker's Specific, 61, 62
Drug addiction, 97, 102, 103. *See also* Cocaine
Drug arrests: and the press, 98–100
    See also Drug laws
Drug education classes, 131
Drug Enforcement Administration, 140
Drug industry, 65–67, 78–79. *See also* Patent medicines
Drug laws, 66, 72, 80, 83, 141, 184–185, 186–187; British, 116, 118; effectiveness of, 65–66, 186–187, 212–214; effects

of, 67, 69–70, 95, 103–104, 144–145, 183–184; federal, 66, 191; institution of, 89–93; state, 190, 191–201, 213, 214. *See also* Anticocaine laws

Drug research, 170–171, 174, 178

Drugs:
acceptance of, by society, 70–73; effects of, 88, 183–184; estimating the amount of use of, 87; prescription, 183. *See also* Alcohol; Amphetamines; Aspirin; Barbiturates; Coca; Cocaine; Heroin; LSD; Marijuana; Methadone; Morphine; Opium; Tranquilizers

Drug use, 13, 15, 97. *See also* Cocaine

Easy Rider, 134
Encyclopédie Méthodique Botanique, 33
Erlenmeyer, Emil, 74, 75
Erythroxyline, 33. *See also* Cocaine
Esquire, 136, 137
Ether, 42
Eye surgery, 42, 43, 44

Fauré, Gabriel, 56
Fauvel, Charles, 43, 56
Federal Bureau of Narcotics, 140
Federal Communications Commission, 134
"Final Problem, The," 54
Finlator, John, 129
First Opium Conference, 1909, 21, 22

Fleischl, Dr., 36, 39, 40, 46, 47, 48
Fonda, Peter, 134
Ford Foundation, Drug Abuse Council of the, 178
Fowler, Gene, 112
French Wine Coca, 59
Freud, Sigmund, 34–41, 48, 51, 71, 180; and cocaine research, 34–41, 42, 44, 45–46, 51, 71, 74, 76, 169, 171
Friedman, Bruce Jay, 137, 138, 139

Gaedecke, 33
Gaedkin, 32
Gibbs, Wolcott, 99
Globe of Flower Cough Syrup, 59
Göring, Herman, 125
Gounod, C. F., 56
Granier-Doyeux, Marcel, 23, 25
Grateful Dead, The, 134
Great American Fraud, The, 79
Gutierrez-Noriega, C., 23, 25

Hague Convention of 1912, 22
Haight-Ashbury Free Medical Clinic, 129
Hallucinogens, 171
Halsted, William Stewart, 46–47
Hammett, Dashiell, 52
Hammond, William, 50
Harrison Narcotics Act, 1914, 66, 91, 93, 99, 102,

104, 107, 116
Harvard Medical School, 77
Hays Office, 111
Heidelberg Ophthalmological
  Society, 44
Heroin, 47, 67, 71, 90, 91,
  111, 119, 126, 127;
  addiction, 28, 48, 95, 129,
  130, 141, 166; prices, 155,
  157; sale of, 93, 145–146
Hitler, Adolf, 125
Hobbes, Thomas, 13
Hodge, William, 16
Holmes, Sherlock, 51, 52,
  53, 54
Hopkins, Jerry, 135, 136
Hopper, Dennis, 134
Hortus Americanus, 16
Hunter, Henry Julian, 131

Inca Empire, 15, 16, 18–21
Indians, Peruvian, 15–21, 27,
  41, 168
International Narcotics Control Board, 23

Jefferson Airplane, 135
Jones, Ernest, 35, 36, 39
*Journal of the American
  Medical Association*, 78,
  82, 134, 135
Jungle, The, 65

Kantner, Paul, 29
King, Pendleton, 94
Koca-Nola, 63
Koch, Christopher, 83
Koller, Karl, 18, 42–43, 44,
  45, 50, 74

"La Coca du Pérou," 57
Lamarck, Jean, 33

Law Enforcement Assistance
  Agency, 87
League of Nations, 21
Leo XIII (pope), 56
Lewin, Louis, 14, 15
Licit & Illicit Drugs, 25, 177
Lindesmith, Alfred, 97, 131
Literature, cocaine in, 51–55,
  94–95, 115–118, 137–139
Louisville Medical News, 34
LSD, 73, 74, 119, 170, 176;
  and alcoholism, 25

McCarthy, Joseph, 84
Mafia. *See* Organized crime
Mantegazza, Paolo, 17
Mariani, Angelo, 55, 56, 57,
  58
Marijuana, 15, 18, 70, 73,
  105, 107, 120, 121, 129,
  144, 176; sources of, 146
Marijuana Tax Act, 1937,
  120–121
Markham, Clement, 17
Massenet, Jules, 56
Mayfield, Curtis, 136
Medical News, 82
Memphis Jug Band, 121
Mescaline, 31
Metcalf's Coca Wine, 60, 61
Methadone, 130, 141, 166
Mitchell, C. L., 62
Modern Times, 110
Monardes, Nicolas, 16
Moreno y Maiz, Thomas,
  34, 43
Morphine, 31, 32, 36, 52,
  59, 67, 71, 76, 80, 88, 89,
  90, 91, 112, 133; addiction,
  39, 47, 51, 58, 75
Mortimer, W. G., 19
Movies, cocaine references

in, 109–110, 111–112, 134, 140

Muscarine, 32

Music, cocaine references in, 109, 110, 134, 135, 136, 140

Musto, David, 131, 132, 134

Mutch, Nathan, 116

Narcotic Drugs Import and Export Act, 1914, 91–92

National Institute on Drug Abuse, 178

Natural History of the Indies, 17

Neil, Fred, 135

Newsweek, 135, 136

New York, magazine, 136,.. 140

New York Times, 84, 89, 98, 102, 129, 140

New York Tribune, 82

Nicotine, 31, 32

Niemann, Albert, 33

"Nightmare of Cocaine, The," 114

Normand, Mabel, 112

Nostrums and Quackery, 63

Nyal's Compound Extract of Damiana, 62

Nyro, Laura, 133

Obersteiner, 74

O'Connor, William A., 122

Olden, Marc, 140

On Morphia Addiction, 75

Opiates, 38, 58, 94, 108. *See also* Opium

Opium, 15, 22, 31, 32, 38, 51, 52, 57, 59, 67, 71, 73, 91; addiction, 75, 76, 77, 80–81; banning of, 90; sale of, 93

Opium Problem, The, 102

Organized crime, and drugs, 152, 153, 154

Paine's Celery Compound, 63, 64

Palmer, Dr., 34

Parke, Davis Company, 67

Patent medicines: cocaine-based, 59–64, 66, 76, 81, 112; industry, 65, 66, 69, 77–79, 91; opium-based, 90; war against, 79–80. *See also* Drug industry

Pellens, Mildred, 131

Pemberton, John Styth, 59

Penfield, Wilder, 46

Penicillin, 48

Peruvian Indians, 15–21, 27, 41, 168

Pharmaceutical Manufacturers' Association, 66

Pharmacologists, 183, 184. *See also* Drug industry

Porter, Cole, 109, 110

Press: coverage of drug arrests, 98–100; reports about cocaine, 110–112, 120–121, 135–137, 139–140

Prohibition: on alcohol, *See* Alcohol; on drugs, *See* Drug laws

Proprietary Association, 66

Proust, Marcel, 115

Psilocybin, 32

Psychopharmacology, 37

"Psychopharmacology of Cocaine, The," 165

Puerto Ricans, in the drug

market, 152
Pure Food and Drug Act, 1906, 63, 65, 66, 79

Quinine, 32

Reefer Madness, 123
Reid, Wallace, 112
Rockefeller, Nelson, 144
Rohmer, Sax, 52, 94
Rolling Stone, 135, 136
Rolling Stones, The, 134, 135
Royal Commentaries of the Incas, 17
Ryno's Hay Fever-n-Catarrh Remedy, 62

Sahm, Doug, 140
"Scandal in Bohemia, A," 51, 53
Schroff, 34, 43
Schultes, Richard Evans, 24
Schultz, Myron, 54, 135
Sertürner, F. W., 32
"Sign of Four, The," 52, 53
Simon, Carleton, 98
Sinclair, Upton, 65, 79
Smith, David, 129
Smith Anti-Cocaine Bill, 1907, 104
Speed. *See* Amphetamines
Spencer, Herbert, 133
Steppenwolf, 135
Stevenson, Robert Louis, 54, 55
Stimmel, H. F., 100–101
Strychnine, 32

Taylor, Desmond, 111
Tea, 14
Terry, Charles, 102, 131
Tobacco, 14

Tranquilizers, 71, 107
Trepanning, 42
Triplex Liver Pills, 59

Uber Coca, 37, 40, 45
United Nations, 21; Commission of Enquiry, 1949, 23; Commission on Narcotics, 1962, 127; Permanent Central Opium Board, 127
U.S. Bureau of Customs, 128
U.S. Congress, 1973 drug report of, 142

Valley of the Dolls, 133
Vanity Fair magazine, 109, 110
Vega, Garcilasso de la, 17
Victoria (queen of England), 56
Vin Mariani, 56, 57, 58
Volstead Act, 108
Von Anrep, 43
Von Tschudi, 17

Watson, Colonel, 83
Weil, Andrew, 183, 224, 225
Welch, William H., 46
White Mountain Press, 137
Wilder, Billy, 134
Wiley, Harvey, 79
Williams, Edward Huntington, 84, 85
Woodley, Richard, 136
Woods, James H., 165
World Health Organization's Expert Committee on Addiction-Producing Drugs, 127

Zinberg, Norman, 177, 208, 223

HELPFUL READING
FROM WARNER BOOKS

SUGAR BLUES
by William Dufty   *(36-181, $3.50)*
Like opium, morphine, and heroin, sugar is an addictive drug, yet Americans consume it daily in everything from cigarettes to bread. If you are overweight, or suffer from migraine, hypoglycemia or acne, the plague of the Sugar Blues has hit you. In fact, by accepted diagnostic standards, *our entire society is pre-diabetic. Sugar Blues* shows you how to live better without it and includes recipes for delicious dishes—all sugar-free!

FOOD, MIND & MOOD
by David Sheinkin, Michael Schachter and
Richard Hutton   *(36-218, $3.50)*
FOOD, MIND & MOOD reveals the simple, easy-to-follow methods of muscle testing, pulse testing and diet control that have restored hundreds of people to happier, healthier lives. Clinically trained psychiatrists Sheinkin and Schachter can help you identify the sources of your problems and regain control of your body and behavior. It could change your life!

EARL MINDELL'S VITAMIN BIBLE
by Earl Mindell   *(L36-174, $3.50)*
Earl Mindell, a certified nutritionist and practicing pharmacist for over fifteen years, heads his own national company specializing in vitamins. His VITAMIN BIBLE is the most comprehensive and complete book about vitamins and nutrient supplements ever written. This important book reveals how vitamin needs vary for each of us and how to determine yours; how to substitute natural substances for tranquilizers, sleeping pills, and other drugs; how the right vitamins can help your heart, retard aging, and improve your sex life.